PUBLIC HEALTH IN THE 21ST CENTURY

ELECTRONIC HEALTH RECORDS

ASSESSMENTS OF PROGRAM PARTICIPATION AND KEY CHALLENGES

PUBLIC HEALTH IN THE 21ST CENTURY

Additional books in this series can be found on Nova's website under the Series tab.

Additional e-books in this series can be found on Nova's website under the e-book tab.

PUBLIC HEALTH IN THE 21ST CENTURY

ELECTRONIC HEALTH RECORDS

ASSESSMENTS OF PROGRAM PARTICIPATION AND KEY CHALLENGES

CAROLE MEDINA
EDITOR

nova publishers
New York

Library of Congress Cataloging-in-Publication Data

ISBN: 978-1-63482-276-3

Published by Nova Science Publishers, Inc. † New York

CONTENTS

Preface vii

Chapter 1 Electronic Health Record Programs: Participation Has Increased, but Action Needed to Achieve Goals, Including Improved Quality of Care 1
United States Government Accountability Office

Chapter 2 Electronic Health Records: HHS Strategy to Address Information Exchange Challenges Lacks Specific Prioritized Actions and Milestones 75
United States Government Accountability Office

Index 113

PREFACE

This book assesses the extent of current and expected participation in the EHR programs; examines information reported by providers and others to measure meaningful use in the EHR programs; evaluates HHS efforts to ensure that EHR data can be reliably used to measure quality of care; and evaluates HHS efforts to assess the effect of the EHR programs on program goals related to adoption and meaningful use of EHRs and improved outcomes.

Chapter 1 - The Health Information Technology for Economic and Clinical Health (HITECH) Act established the EHR programs, which provide incentive payments for—and later are expected to apply penalties to—certain providers, such as hospitals and professionals, to encourage them to demonstrate meaningful use of certified EHR technology and meet other program requirements. For example, one measure of meaningful use requires providers to implement checks for potential drug interactions with patients' other drugs and allergies.

As mandated by the HITECH Act, GAO (1) assessed the extent of current and expected participation in the EHR programs, (2) examined information reported by providers and others to measure meaningful use in the EHR programs, (3) evaluated HHS efforts to ensure that EHR data can be reliably used to measure quality of care, and (4) evaluated HHS efforts to assess the effect of the EHR programs on program goals related to adoption and meaningful use of EHRs and improved outcomes. GAO analyzed data from CMS and other sources; reviewed applicable statutes, regulations, and guidance; and interviewed officials from HHS and stakeholder groups.

Chapter 2 - The Health Information Technology for Economic and Clinical Health Act (HITECH) promotes the use of health information technology and identifies the importance of health information exchange. It provides incentive payments to promote the widespread adoption and meaningful use of EHR technology. To be a meaningful user, providers are to demonstrate, among other things, that their certified EHR technology can electronically exchange health information. GAO examined (1) the key challenges to the electronic exchange of health information, if any, that have been reported by providers and stakeholders, and HHS's ongoing efforts to address them, and (2) the extent to which HHS has planned future actions to address those key challenges. GAO reviewed HHS documentation; interviewed HHS officials; and interviewed providers— hospital officials and physicians—and relevant stakeholders about their experiences.

In: Electronic Health Records
Editor: Carole Medina
ISBN: 978-1-63482-276-3

Chapter 1

ELECTRONIC HEALTH RECORD PROGRAMS: PARTICIPATION HAS INCREASED, BUT ACTION NEEDED TO ACHIEVE GOALS, INCLUDING IMPROVED QUALITY OF CARE*

United States Government Accountability Office

WHY GAO DID THIS STUDY

The Health Information Technology for Economic and Clinical Health (HITECH) Act established the EHR programs, which provide incentive payments for—and later are expected to apply penalties to—certain providers, such as hospitals and professionals, to encourage them to demonstrate meaningful use of certified EHR technology and meet other program requirements. For example, one measure of meaningful use requires providers to implement checks for potential drug interactions with patients' other drugs and allergies.

As mandated by the HITECH Act, GAO (1) assessed the extent of current and expected participation in the EHR programs, (2) examined information reported by providers and others to measure meaningful use in the EHR programs, (3) evaluated HHS efforts to ensure that EHR data can be reliably

---

* This is an edited, reformatted and augmented version of a United States Government Accountability Office publication, No. GAO-14-207, dated March 2014.

used to measure quality of care, and (4) evaluated HHS efforts to assess the effect of the EHR programs on program goals related to adoption and meaningful use of EHRs and improved outcomes. GAO analyzed data from CMS and other sources; reviewed applicable statutes, regulations, and guidance; and interviewed officials from HHS and stakeholder groups.

What GAO Recommends

GAO recommends that HHS develop a comprehensive strategy to better ensure the reliability of CQM data collected using EHRs and develop and use outcome-oriented performance measures to monitor progress toward goals. HHS agreed data reliability and performance monitoring are important but neither agreed nor disagreed with GAO's recommendations.

What GAO Found

Based on the number of providers awarded incentive payments, participation in the Department of Health and Human Services' (HHS) Medicare and Medicaid Electronic Health Record (EHR) programs increased substantially from their first year in 2011 to 2012. For hospitals, participation increased from 45 percent of those eligible for 2011 to 64 percent of those eligible for 2012. For professionals, such as physicians, participation increased from 21 percent of those eligible for 2011 to 48 percent of those eligible for 2012. While increases occurred, a substantial percentage of providers that participated in 2011 did not participate in 2012. Officials who oversee the programs at the Centers for Medicare & Medicaid Services (CMS) noted there could be several reasons for this, such as challenges in demonstrating meaningful use, and are monitoring the issue. Various program changes make future participation difficult to estimate. For example, increased stringency of requirements for the programs' second phase beginning in 2014—Stage 2—may slow participation, while the introduction of penalties in 2015 for some providers may motivate participation.

Reporting on meaningful use for 2011 and 2012 indicates that providers who have already participated in the programs' first phase—Stage 1—used their certified EHR systems more often than required. For example, for both 2011 and 2012, Medicare hospitals reported using computerized provider order entry for over 84 percent of patients—in excess of the required threshold for Stage 1 of 30 percent. However, some meaningful use measures may be more challenging for providers, including measures involving the electronic exchange of information. For example, less than 15 percent of professionals reported on an optional Stage 1 measure to provide a summary of care document at each care transition or referral, which is mandatory in Stage 2. A CMS official said the agency is taking steps to help providers prepare for Stage 2 meaningful use measures.

The lack of a comprehensive strategy limits HHS's ability to ensure the department can reliably use the clinical quality measures (CQM) collected in certified EHRs for quality measurement activities. Reliability issues persist, although CMS and HHS's Office of the National Coordinator for Health Information Technology (ONC) have made efforts to address concerns. For example, different providers may report CQMs based on and tested to different requirements depending on whether their EHRs have incorporated technical updates. Without a comprehensive strategy, efforts to address reliability issues (in accordance with the internal control standard requiring relevant and reliable information) and improve quality and efficiency may be limited.

Consistent with law and GAO guidance on assessing agency performance, HHS, CMS, and ONC have established some performance measures for the EHR programs that are tied to strategic goals regarding adoption and meaningful use of EHRs; however, they have not established measures that would help them to track progress toward program outcomes such as health care quality, efficiency, and patient safety. Although HHS expects that the use of EHRs can help achieve improved outcomes and support other efforts that are also intended to improve care, that result is not yet assured. CMS and ONC may lack critical information necessary to establish program priorities and subsequently make program adjustments based on progress toward outcomes.

ABBREVIATIONS

CHIME	College of Healthcare Information Management Executives
CMS	Centers for Medicare & Medicaid Services
CQM	clinical quality measure
EHR	electronic health record
GPRAMA	Government Performance and Results Act Modernization Act of 2010
HHS	Department of Health and Human Services

HIT	health information technology
HITECH	Act Health Information Technology for Economic and Clinical Health Act
IQR	Inpatient Quality Reporting
ONC	Office of the National Coordinator for Health Information Technology
PQRS	Physician Quality Reporting System

* * *

March 6, 2014

Congressional Committees

The Medicare and Medicaid Electronic Health Record (EHR) programs began in 2011 with a goal of promoting the adoption and meaningful use of certified EHR technology.[1] As of 2009, before the programs began, studies estimated that 78 percent of office-based physicians and 91 percent of hospitals had not adopted EHRs.[2] Such technology has the potential to improve the quality of care patients receive and to reduce health care costs, if the technology is used in a way that improves providers' and patients' access to critical information. The Medicare and Medicaid EHR programs are the largest of the activities, in terms of potential federal expenditures, and are funded by the Health Information Technology for Economic and Clinical Health (HITECH) Act, which was enacted as part of the American Recovery and Reinvestment Act of 2009 and provides funding for various activities to promote the adoption and meaningful use of certified EHR technology.[3] The Congressional Budget Office estimated total spending for these activities to be $30 billion from 2011 through 2019.[4]

To increase the adoption and meaningful use of certified EHR technology, the Medicare and Medicaid EHR programs provide incentive payments for providers—that is, certain types of hospitals, such as critical access hospitals, and certain types of professionals, such as physicians and nurse practitioners.[5] Additionally, beginning in 2015, the Medicare EHR program is to begin applying a payment adjustment, referred to in this report as a penalty, for hospitals and professionals that treat Medicare patients but do not meet the Medicare EHR program requirements.[6] In establishing the EHR programs, Congress defined "a meaningful EHR user" as a hospital or professional that meets the following three criteria: (1) demonstrates use of certified EHR technology in a meaningful manner; (2) demonstrates that certified EHR technology is connected in a manner that provides for the electronic exchange of health information to improve the quality of health care, such as promoting care coordination; and (3) uses certified EHR technology to submit information on clinical quality measures (CQM) and other measures.[7] The EHR programs were designed to last for multiple years to increase, over time, the widespread adoption and meaningful use of EHRs, which is viewed by the Department of Health and Human Services (HHS) and others as a necessary step toward transforming health care into a system that can achieve goals of improved quality, efficiency, and patient safety. For example, use of EHRs could improve efficiency by reducing the duplication of diagnostic tests, or improve patient safety by preventing medical errors resulting from, for example, incomplete medical histories for new patients. Additionally, CQM data collected by providers using EHRs could be used by HHS to measure and improve health care quality by, for example, designing programs that compensate providers for meeting quality and efficiency targets—that is, pay for performance.

Within HHS, the Centers for Medicare & Medicaid Services (CMS) and the Office of the National Coordinator for Health Information Technology (ONC) have developed the EHR programs' requirements.[8] CMS is responsible for administering the Medicare EHR program and overseeing and funding most of the Medicaid EHR program, which is administered by the states and U.S. insular areas.[9] ONC is responsible for overseeing the certification of EHR technology, including establishing technical standards and certification criteria for it.[10] Additionally, ONC is charged with formulating the federal government's health information technology (HIT) strategy and coordinating federal HIT policies, programs, and investments.[11]

The HITECH Act requires us to report on the effect of the act on a number of important areas.[12] Our work has focused on the Medicare and Medicaid EHR programs because of the potential magnitude of federal expenditures for those programs. In April 2012 we reported on CMS's efforts to oversee the Medicare EHR program during its first year as well as challenges encountered by providers and strategies they used to participate in the program.[13] We recommended that CMS take steps to enhance its processes to verify that providers met the requirements to receive incentive payments. On behalf of CMS, HHS agreed with most of our recommendations. In July 2012 we reported information on providers that were awarded Medicare EHR incentive payments for 2011, including the number of award recipients and their characteristics.[14] In December 2012 we reported information on providers that were awarded Medicaid EHR incentive payments for 2011, including the number of award recipients and their characteristics.[15] In October 2013 we reported information on providers that were awarded Medicare EHR incentive payments for 2011 and 2012, including the number of award recipients and their characteristics.[16] Ongoing work is examining the key challenges to the electronic exchange of health information that have been reported by providers and stakeholders and HHS's efforts to address those challenges. In this report, we (1) assess the extent of current and expected participation in the EHR programs; (2) examine information reported by providers and others to measure meaningful use in the EHR programs; (3) evaluate HHS's efforts to ensure that EHR data can be reliably used to measure quality of care; and (4) evaluate HHS's efforts to assess the effect of the EHR programs on program goals related to adoption and meaningful use of EHRs and improved outcomes such as quality, efficiency, and patient safety. In addition, the HITECH Act specified that we report on the effect of the act on, among other things, health insurance premiums, and such information is provided in appendix I.

To assess the extent of current participation in the Medicare and Medicaid EHR programs, we analyzed data related to the 2011 and 2012 program years that CMS collected in its National Level Repository through October 23, 2013.[17] Using these data, we

- estimated the percentage of eligible providers awarded a Medicare or Medicaid (or both) EHR incentive payment for 2011 and for 2012;
- determined the total amount of Medicare and Medicaid EHR incentive payments awarded to providers each year; and
- estimated the percentage of providers that were awarded a Medicare or Medicaid (or, in the case of some hospitals, both) EHR incentive payment for 2011 but not for 2012.[18]

To assess the extent of expected participation in the EHR programs, we interviewed CMS officials regarding agency activities to increase participation and efforts to ensure that providers continue to participate in the EHR programs after their first year. We also interviewed individuals from organizations representing stakeholders, including the American Hospital Association and the College of Healthcare Information Management Executives (CHIME), whose members include health care chief information officers; and reviewed an analysis of 2012 survey data of hospitals collected by the American Hospital Association. In addition, we reviewed applicable regulations and other relevant agency documents.

To examine information reported by providers and others to measure meaningful use in the EHR programs, we analyzed data CMS collected in its National Level Repository through October 23, 2013. Specifically, we analyzed data that providers reported to CMS for the 2011 and 2012 program years to demonstrate meaningful use under the Medicare EHR program—known as meaningful use measures. We analyzed the CMS data to identify

- the extent to which providers exceeded reporting thresholds, which are specified percentages of patients or actions that providers must meet or exceed to satisfy the requirements of a subset of the meaningful use measures (14 hospital measures and 16 professional measures); and
- the frequency with which providers reported meaningful use measures without claiming exemptions, which are allowed under the program for some measures if providers meet certain criteria specific to the individual measures (e.g., the measure is not relevant to their patient populations or clinical practices, the providers conducted too few actions to be measured, or the providers were not able to perform the action).[19]

As part of our analysis, we also reviewed a CMS analysis of meaningful use measure data submitted by professionals to states to demonstrate meaningful use in the Medicaid EHR program for the 2012 program year, reviewed an analysis of 2012 survey data of hospitals collected by the American Hospital Association, and analyzed 2012 survey data collected by the National Center for Health Statistics in the Centers for Disease Control and Prevention from office-based physicians. We identified meaningful use measures related to electronic health information exchange based on information obtained from officials from CMS and ONC. We interviewed officials from CMS, ONC, the American Hospital Association, the American Medical Association, and CHIME, and reviewed letters submitted by stakeholder organizations to HHS related to the EHR programs. In addition, we reviewed regulations and other relevant agency documentation.

To evaluate HHS's efforts to ensure that EHR data can be reliably used to measure quality of care, we reviewed letters submitted by stakeholder organizations to HHS related to the EHR programs; reviewed the EHR programs' requirements and agency documentation describing HHS's quality measurement activities, including the Inpatient Prospective Payment System and the Physician Fee Schedule regulations; reviewed other materials related to quality measurement; and interviewed officials from CMS, ONC, the American Hospital Association, and CHIME.[20] We also reviewed relevant internal control standards regarding information used by agencies and compared them against HHS activities.[21] We analyzed CQM data that providers reported to CMS to demonstrate meaningful use under the Medicare EHR program for the 2011 and 2012 program years and that are captured in CMS's National Level Repository. Specifically, we analyzed the extent to which Medicare providers had few patients who could be included in the calculation of at least one clinical quality measure.[22]

To ensure the reliability of the various data we analyzed, we interviewed officials from CMS, reviewed relevant documentation, and conducted electronic testing to identify missing data and obvious errors. On the basis of these activities, we determined that the data were sufficiently reliable for our analysis. (For more information on our data analysis, see app. II.)

To evaluate HHS's efforts to assess the effect of the EHR programs on program goals, we reviewed HHS's Fiscal Years 2010-2015 Strategic Plan, ONC's 2011-2015 Federal Health Information Technology Strategic Plan, and the EHR programs' requirements to identify department and agency goals particularly relevant to the EHR programs. We also reviewed HHS's Fiscal Year 2014 Annual Performance Report and Performance Plan, CMS's Fiscal Year 2014 Budget Justification, and ONC's Fiscal Year 2014 Budget Justification to identify department and agency performance measures relevant to the EHR programs. In addition, we interviewed CMS and ONC officials regarding performance measures and program evaluations relevant to the EHR programs. We assessed this evidence against relevant criteria from the Government Performance and Results Act Modernization Act of 2010 (GPRAMA) as incorporated in our guidance on assessing performance and our guidance on designing evaluations.[23]

We conducted this performance audit from February 2013 through March 2014 in accordance with generally accepted government auditing standards. Those standards require that we plan and perform the audit to obtain sufficient, appropriate evidence to provide a reasonable basis for our findings and conclusions based on our audit objectives. We believe that the evidence obtained provides a reasonable basis for our findings and conclusions based on our audit objectives.

Background

Incentive Payments and Penalties

Through use of incentive payments and penalties, the EHR programs are intended to help address the significant barriers to the adoption and use of EHRs, such as cost, and the technical challenges associated with their use. Beginning in 2011, the first year of the Medicare and Medicaid EHR programs, the programs have provided incentive payments to participating providers, that is, eligible providers that met program requirements.[24] Beginning in 2015, CMS is generally required to begin applying a penalty to hospitals and professionals that do not meet the Medicare EHR program requirements. There is no statutory end-point provided for the penalties. The Medicaid EHR program does not impose penalties on Medicaid providers that do not meet the Medicaid EHR program's requirements by a specific date; however, if Medicaid providers also treat Medicare patients, they are required to meet the Medicare EHR program's requirements from 2015 onward to avoid penalties from the Medicare EHR program. (See fig. 1.)

The amount of incentive payment varies depending on the type of provider (hospital or professional) and the program in which the provider participates (Medicare EHR program or Medicaid EHR program). For most hospitals, the incentive payment amount for any given year is generally based on the hospital's annual discharges and Medicare share (i.e., percentage of the hospital's inpatient bed days that were attributable to Medicare patients) for the Medicare EHR program, or Medicaid share (i.e., percentage of the hospital's inpatient bed days that were attributable to Medicaid patients) for the Medicaid EHR program.[25] However, for critical access hospitals in the Medicare EHR program, the incentive payment amount is generally based on the hospital's Medicare share as well as the reasonable costs incurred for the purchase of depreciable assets necessary to administer certified EHR technology, such as computers and associated hardware and software. Professionals in the Medicare EHR program generally cannot earn more than $18,000 in incentive payments in their first year, and total payments cannot exceed $44,000.[26] In the Medicaid EHR program, professionals cannot earn more than $21,250 in incentive payments in the first year, and total payments cannot exceed $63,750.

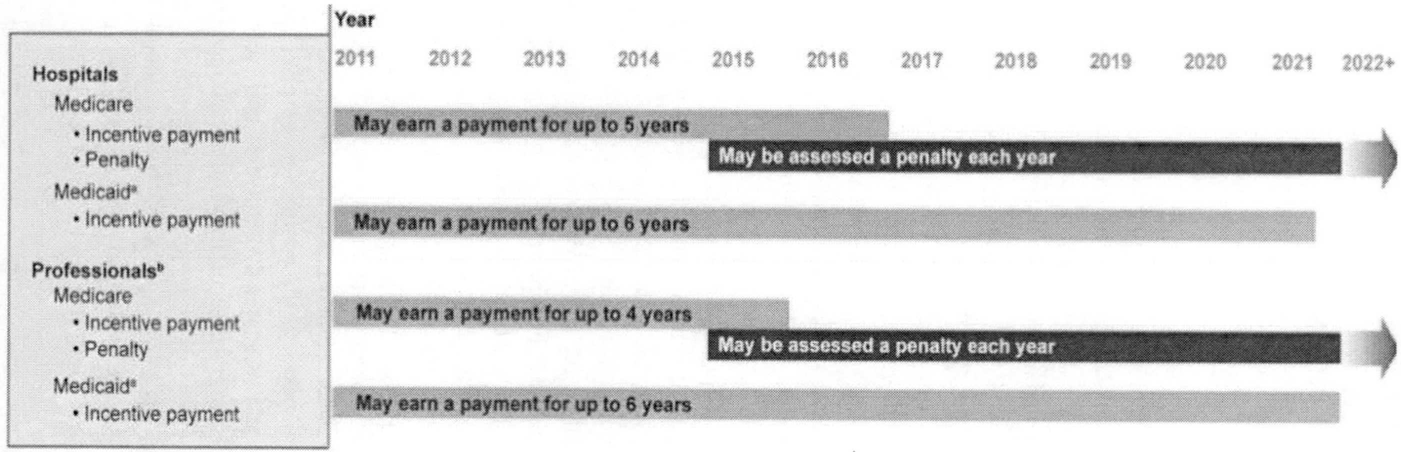

Source: Health Information Technology for Economic and Clinical Health Act.

Notes: Program years are determined and awarded on a fiscal year basis for hospitals and on a calendar year basis for professionals. Professionals may not receive incentive payments under both the Medicare EHR program and the Medicaid EHR program during the same year; they must choose one of the two programs under which they will participate. In contrast, hospitals may qualify for incentive payments under both programs during the same year.

[a]If Medicaid providers also treat Medicare patients, they are required to meet the Medicare EHR program's requirements from 2015 onward to avoid penalties from the Medicare EHR program.

In the Medicare and Medicaid EHR programs, professionals include doctors of medicine and dental surgery. In the Medicaid EHR program, professionals also include nurse practitioners, certified nurse-midwives, and certain physician assistants.

Figure 1. Years in Which Incentive Payments Are Available and When Penalties Will Be Assessed in the Medicare and Medicaid Electronic Health Record (EHR) Programs.

Beginning in 2015, CMS will apply penalties to Medicare providers if they did not meet Medicare EHR program requirements. [27] For most hospitals, penalties will be applied by reducing the Medicare Inpatient Prospective Payment System payment rate increase by 25 percent each year, with a maximum cumulative reduction of 75 percent.[28] However, for critical access hospitals, the penalty is applicable to the hospital's Medicare reimbursement for inpatient services. For professionals, penalties will be assessed by reducing the reimbursement that the provider would ordinarily receive for furnishing Medicare Part B services by 1 percent for each year the professional did not meet the requirements, with a cumulative penalty of up to 3 percent per year.[29] CMS may exempt hospitals and professionals from penalties if it determines that complying with the program requirements would result in a significant hardship to the provider; such exemptions are to be granted on a case-by-case basis subject to annual renewal.[30] Examples of permissible hardship circumstances include lacking necessary infrastructure, such as internet broadband; facing unforeseen circumstances such as a natural disaster; or, for professionals, lacking patient interaction.

Medicare EHR Program and Medicaid EHR Program Requirements

CMS has established requirements for the EHR programs that specify the providers eligible to participate—that is, providers that are permitted to earn incentive payments or that may be subject to penalties. For example, providers must be a permissible provider type, such as an acute care hospital or a doctor of medicine and, for the Medicaid EHR program, providers must generally meet a patient volume requirement to be eligible.[31] In addition to meeting program eligibility requirements, to receive incentive payments or avoid penalties, eligible providers must also satisfy reporting requirements by submitting information to CMS for the Medicare EHR program, to the states for the Medicaid EHR program, or to both. The reporting requirements generally incorporate the three statutory criteria for "meaningful use" established in HITECH—(1) demonstrate use of certified EHR technology in a meaningful manner; (2) demonstrate that certified EHR technology is connected in a manner that provides for the electronic exchange of health information; and (3) submit information on CQMs using certified EHR technology. To receive incentive payments from the Medicare EHR program, the information reported by providers must satisfy all three statutory criteria;

that is, providers must “demonstrate meaningful use.” However, to receive incentive payments from the Medicaid EHR program in their first year of participation, providers need not satisfy the three statutory criteria. Instead, they must only report that they adopted, implemented, or upgraded to certified EHR technology.[32] In subsequent years, though, they must demonstrate meaningful use to receive incentive payments.

Certified EHR Technology

Certified EHR technology is technology that has been determined by ONC-authorized organizations—referred to as certification bodies and testing laboratories—to conform to the standards and certification criteria developed by ONC. ONC has changed the certification criteria since the EHR programs began. Specifically, providers who participated in the EHR programs from 2011 through 2013 were generally required to use 2011-edition EHRs and all providers who participate in the EHR programs from 2014 through 2016—regardless of whether the provider participated in the program in earlier years—are required to use 2014-edition EHRs. [33] ONC is expected to develop another set of certification criteria for EHRs that providers would be required to use beginning in 2017.[34]

Meaningful Use Measures

These measures are intended to promote the use of EHRs in the delivery of health care and to ensure that providers capture information in their EHRs consistently. For example, one measure requires providers to enable a technical capability of their EHRs to notify the provider of potential interactions among the patients’ medications and with patients’ allergies. Providers must report certain mandatory measures and also must report a set of optional measures that they may choose from a menu. The meaningful use measures are being implemented in three stages that will apply to different providers in different years.[35] This approach is consistent with the HITECH Act, which directed the Secretary of HHS to seek to improve health care quality and the use of EHRs by requiring more stringent requirements over time. According to CMS, using the staged approach is intended to help overcome two important deficiencies—the lack of widespread use of capable EHRs and the lack of an HIT infrastructure—that existed when the requirements were being developed, with the hope that those deficiencies would be addressed over time as a result of the EHR programs. The stage that is applicable to each provider in each year is based on the first year in which the provider demonstrated meaningful use in the Medicare EHR program or the Medicaid EHR program. For example, a Medicare professional that first demonstrated meaningful use in 2011 must report the Stage 1 meaningful use measures for 2011, 2012, and 2013 to receive incentive payments for those years and must report the Stage 2 meaningful use measures beginning in 2014 to receive an incentive payment for that year.[36] The Stage 3 requirements have not yet been developed but are expected to be finalized in 2015 and to apply beginning in 2017. (See table 1.)

Table 1. Stages of Meaningful Use Measures

First year provider demonstrates meaningful use[a]	Stage of measures (•Stage 1; ••Stage 2; •••Stage 3)							
	2011	2012	2013	2014	2015	2016	2017	2018
2011	•	•	•	••	••	••	•••	[b]
2012		•	•	••	••	••	•••	[b]
2013			•	•	••	••	•••	•••
2014				•	•	••	••	•••
2015					•	•	••	••
2016						•	•	••
2017							•	•

Source: CMS.

Notes: Providers participating in the Medicare Electronic Health Record (EHR) program are subject to the stage of meaningful use measures as indicated above even if they stop participating in one year and resume in a later year. For example, if a Medicare provider first demonstrated meaningful use in 2012 but did not participate in the Medicare EHR program again until 2014, that provider would be required to report the Stage 2 measures in 2014, 2015, and 2016. However, this is not the case for providers participating in the Medicaid EHR program. Instead, a Medicaid provider that first demonstrated meaningful use in 2012 but did not participate in the Medicaid EHR program again until 2014 would be required to report the Stage 1 measures in 2014 and the Stage 2 measures in 2015. Except for 2014, providers must collect data related to the meaningful use measures in any 90 consecutive days in their first year of reporting meaningful use and for a full year in subsequent years. For 2014 only, all providers, regardless of their stage of meaningful use, are only required to collect data related to the meaningful use measures for 3 months.

[a]The table assumes Medicaid providers' first year of participation is for adopting, implementing, or upgrading to a certified EHR system and that those providers participate in consecutive years.

[b]CMS has not yet determined whether additional meaningful use stages will be developed or when those would apply.

The meaningful use measures in Stage 1 are intended to promote the electronic capture of health information in a structured format and to encourage providers to use that information to track key clinical conditions. The Stage 2 meaningful use measures were chosen to encourage continuous quality improvement at the point of care and are more stringent than the Stage 1 measures. For example, measures that were formerly optional are now mandatory, and some measures require that the provider perform the action for a greater percentage of patients or implement more interventions. Additionally, ONC and CMS have stated that Stage 2 places a stronger emphasis on electronic health information exchange with other providers compared to Stage 1.[37] CMS has stated its intention to develop even more stringent meaningful use measures for Stage 3 that would promote activities that can lead to improved health outcomes, such as using decision support tools or providing patient access to self-management tools.

Table 2 provides information on the number and type of measures that providers must report for Stage 1 and Stage 2.

Table 2. Numbers of Meaningful Use Measures by Stage

Provider		Stage 1[a]	Stage 2
Hospitals	Mandatory	14	16
	Optional	5 of 10 menu	3 of 6 menu
	Total	19	19
Professionals	Mandatory	15	17
	Optional	5 of 10 menu	3 of 6 menu
	Total	20	20

Source: CMS.

Note: For a list of the meaningful use measures by stage, see appendix III.

[a]CMS made changes to the Stage 1 requirements that apply after 2012 which are not reflected in this table.

Clinical Quality Measures (CQM)

Health care quality measures, also known as CQMs, can be used to assess provider performance and to drive quality improvement and accountability. For example, one CQM for professionals measures the use of high-risk medications in the elderly. CQMs are composed of a number of clinical data elements, or pieces of data, that must be collected in order to determine performance on any given measure. Using those data elements, a score for the measure can then be calculated. [38] In order to demonstrate meaningful use in the Medicare or Medicaid EHR programs, providers are required to collect CQMs electronically using EHRs and report those data to CMS (Medicare), the states (Medicaid), or both. However, historically, CQMs have been collected through other data collection methods, such as through a detailed, manual review of paper medical records, a process referred to as chart abstraction. Most of the CQMs identified by CMS for use in the EHR programs were originally developed for paper medical records or other data collection methods and later modified so they could be collected using EHRs.[39]

The CQMs that providers must collect using EHRs and report to demonstrate meaningful use are determined by the edition of certified EHRs providers must use. Specifically, using their 2011-edition certified EHRs that applied from 2011 to 2013, hospitals were required to report all 15 CQMs identified by CMS, and professionals were required to report 6 CQMs from a list of 44 measures.[40] Using their 2014-edition certified EHRs that will apply from 2014 to 2016, hospitals are required to report 16 CQMs from a list of 29 measures, and professionals are required to report 9 CQMs from a list of 64 measures.[41] Medicare providers are being encouraged to electronically report the results of CQMs to CMS, but they have the option of reporting CQMs by manually entering information into CMS's web-based tools, a process known as attestation.[42]

HHS's Quality Measurement Activities

In addition to the EHR programs, HHS requires providers to collect and report CQMs for a number of other programs in order to measure health care quality, some of which provide financial incentives to health care providers to help achieve the goals of improved quality and efficiency. For example, CMS is to impose penalties on providers who do not satisfactorily report quality data to the Hospital Inpatient Quality Reporting (IQR) program and to the Physician Quality Reporting System (PQRS). The Patient Protection and Affordable Care Act directed HHS to implement new programs that will use CQMs, including pay-forperformance programs such as the Physician Value Based Payment Modifier program, which bases Medicare payments in part on CQM results, and the Medicare Shared Savings Program, which rewards Accountable Care Organizations that lower growth in health care costs while meeting performance standards.[43]

Across its programs, HHS has a goal to use CQMs that are broad based, patient centered, and prioritized based on their potential to achieve population-wide improvements. In order to do this in its programs, CMS has set a goal of collecting and submitting data using EHRs, which HHS officials have indicated can be used to collect CQMs as a byproduct of the routine delivery of health care. To minimize the burden on providers of collecting and reporting similar CQMs for different CMS programs using differing methods, CMS has modified some of its programs' requirements such that providers may submit data collected through EHRs as part of the Medicare or Medicaid EHR programs instead of separately collecting and submitting data through other methods such as chart abstraction. For example,

- Hospitals electronically reporting to CMS one-quarter of CQM data collected in 2014 using 2014-edition EHRs for 16 CQMs will satisfy the IQR program's four-quarter reporting requirement for those 16 measures for 2016 payment determinations and the Medicare EHR program's CQM reporting requirement for 2014.[44]
- Professionals electronically reporting one year of CQM data generated from 2014-edition EHRs to CMS for PQRS in 2014 will satisfy the CQM reporting requirements for both PQRS and the Medicare EHR program.[45] CMS will use those data for professionals in practices of 10 or more individuals to generate the Physician Value Based Payment Modifier that will be applied to payments made under the Medicare physician fee schedule starting January 1, 2016.[46]

Performance Assessment

GPRAMA requires federal agencies to prepare performance reports and establish performance measures to assess performance of federal programs. Performance measures assess performance via ongoing monitoring and reporting of program accomplishments, which include progress toward pre-established goals. Our previous work notes that performance measures can serve as an early warning system to management and as a vehicle for improving accountability to the public.[47] We have also published guidance on assessing performance that incorporates GPRAMA criteria and which states that it is important for performance measures to be tied to program goals and for agencies to ensure their activities support their organizational missions and move them closer to accomplishing their strategic goals.[48] In addition, our guidance to federal agencies on designing evaluations suggests that performance measures should include both process and outcome measures (see table 3).[49] Outcome measures are particularly useful in assessing the status of program operations, identifying areas that need improvement, and ensuring accountability for end results. Furthermore, our guidance on assessing performance notes that leading organizations not only establish performance measures but also use information from these performance measures to continuously improve processes, identify program priorities, and set improvement goals.

Table 3. Description of Process and Outcome Measures

Type of measure	Description	Example
Process	Addresses the type or level of program activities conducted and the direct products or services delivered by a program	The number of participants enrolled in a job training program
Outcome	Addresses the results of products and services	The percentage of participants who find employment after successfully completing the job training program

Source: GAO.

PARTICIPATION IN THE EHR PROGRAMS HAS INCREASED, BUT PROGRAM CHANGES MAKE IT DIFFICULT TO ESTIMATE FUTURE PARTICIPATION

Participation in CMS's EHR programs increased substantially from 2011 to 2012, but some providers who participated in 2011 did not continue in 2012. It is difficult to estimate future participation in the EHR programs because of various program changes, including the planned increase in stringency of the meaningful use measures, the introduction of penalties for some providers in 2015, CMS's efforts to increase participation among certain providers, and changes to eligibility requirements.

Participation in 2012 Increased Even Though Some Providers Did Not Continue after 2011

Participation in CMS's EHR programs increased substantially from 2011 to 2012.[50] For hospitals, participation increased from 45 percent of those eligible for 2011 to 64 percent of those eligible for 2012.[51] For professionals, participation increased from 21 percent of those eligible for 2011 to 48 percent of those eligible for 2012.[52] (See fig. 2.)

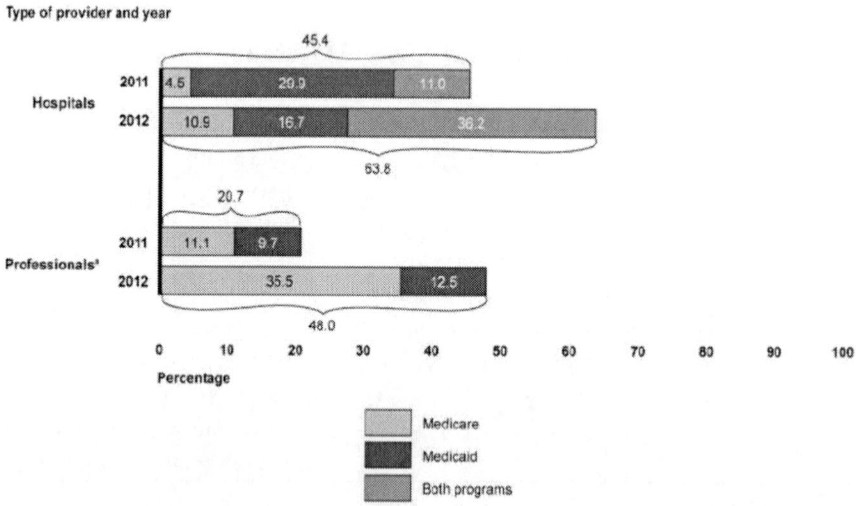

Source: GAO analysis of CMS data.

Notes: We analyzed data CMS collected pertaining to the EHR programs through October 23, 2013. This figure illustrates the percentage of eligible providers awarded EHR program incentive payments for 2011 and for 2012, as indicated by the length of each bar. As designated by the legend, these bars are divided to indicate the percentage of eligible providers that were awarded an incentive payment for the Medicare EHR program or the Medicaid EHR program or, in the case of hospitals, both EHR programs. These figures do not include participation in the Medicare Advantage EHR program. The sums of the percentages listed by EHR program may not equal the percentage reported for the entire year due to rounding. We estimated the percentage of eligible providers awarded incentive payments by dividing the number of providers awarded incentive payments by the total number of eligible providers CMS estimated in its Stage 1 final rule. Specifically, CMS estimated that 5,013 hospitals and 521,600 professionals were eligible for the Medicare or Medicaid EHR program 2011 and 5,013 hospitals and 527,200 professionals for 2012.

[a]In the Medicare and Medicaid EHR programs, professionals include doctors of medicine and dental surgery. In the Medicaid EHR program, professionals also include nurse practitioners, certified nurse-midwives, and certain physician assistants.

Figure 2. Percentage of Eligible Hospitals and Professionals Participating in the Electronic Health Record (EHR) Programs, 2011 and 2012.

The amount CMS paid in incentive payments to providers for participating in the Medicare EHR program, Medicaid EHR program, or both programs increased from $5.2 billion for 2011 to $9.5 billion for 2012.[53] In total, CMS paid $14.7 billion in incentive payments to providers for 2011 and 2012.[54] Of this total, hospitals received nearly $8.6 billion and professionals received almost $6.1 billion. Incentive payments for hospitals and professionals under the Medicare EHR program amounted to $8.8 billion, while incentive payments for hospitals and professionals under the Medicaid EHR program were $5.9 billion. (See fig. 3.)

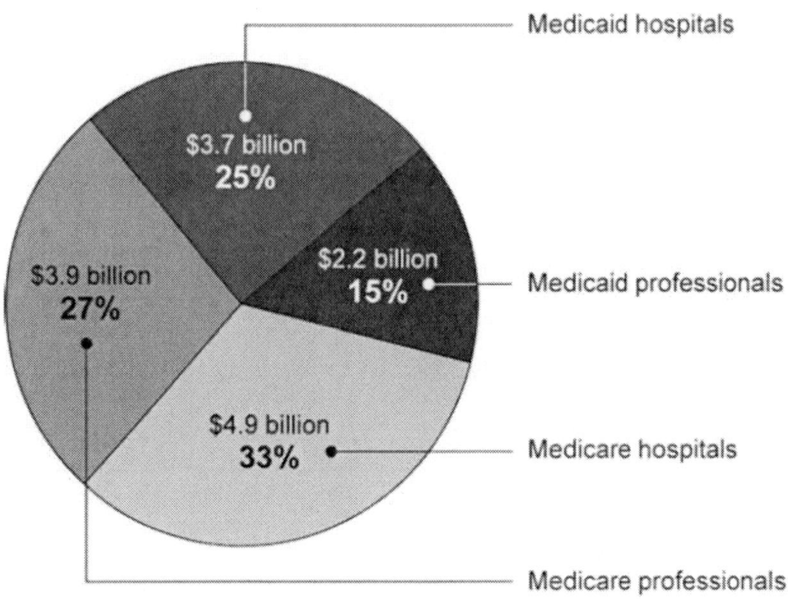

Source: GAO analysis of CMS data.

Notes: We analyzed data CMS collected pertaining to the EHR programs through October 23, 2013. These figures do not include participation in the Medicare Advantage EHR program. In the Medicare and Medicaid EHR programs, professionals include doctors of medicine and dental surgery.

In the Medicaid EHR program, professionals also include nurse practitioners, certified nurse-midwives, and certain physician assistants.

Figure 3. Total Payments from the Electronic Health Record (EHR) Programs for 2011 and 2012, by Program and Provider Type.

Although participation in the EHR programs has increased overall, a substantial percentage of providers that participated in the Medicare EHR program or Medicaid EHR program in 2011 did not participate in either program in 2012. (See fig. 4.) Specifically, within the 36 states that had completed their determinations of which providers would receive incentive payments for the 2012 Medicaid EHR program year, 61 percent of professionals and 36 percent of hospitals that participated in the Medicaid EHR program in 2011 did not continue in 2012.[55] Sixteen percent of professionals and 10 percent of hospitals participating in the Medicare EHR program in 2011 did not continue to participate in 2012.

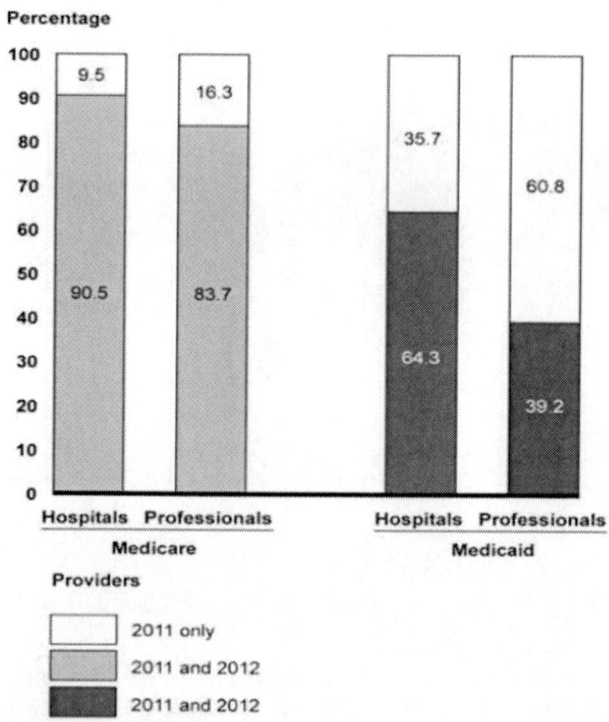

Source: GAO analysis of CMS data.

Notes: We analyzed data CMS collected pertaining to the EHR programs through October 23, 2013.

The information presented for Medicaid providers is based on an analysis of data for 36 states that, according to CMS, had completed their determinations of which providers would receive incentive payments for the 2011 and 2012 Medicaid EHR program years as of October 23, 2013. The "2011 and 2012" bars include providers that switched between participating in the Medicare EHR program in 2011 and the Medicaid EHR program in 2012, or vice versa. In the Medicare and Medicaid EHR programs, professionals include doctors of medicine and dental surgery. In the Medicaid EHR program, professionals also include nurse practitioners, certified nurse-midwives, and certain physician assistants.

Figure 4. Percentage of 2011 Electronic Health Record (EHR) Programs Participants, by Participation in 2011 Alone or in Both 2011 and 2012.

CMS officials are aware that some providers participating in 2011 did not continue in 2012 and told us that they are monitoring the issue and taking steps to reverse this trend. One CMS official told us there are various possible reasons Medicare and Medicaid providers did not continue to participate in the EHR programs. Noteworthy for the Medicaid EHR program, and in contrast to the Medicare EHR program, providers do not need to participate in consecutive years to maximize their incentive payments, and there are no penalties for not participating. Another possible reason providers did not continue to participate in the Medicaid EHR program in 2012 is that providers are not required to demonstrate meaningful use for their first year of participation, but must do so for their second year. One CMS official noted that a provider who received an incentive payment for adopting, implementing, or upgrading to a certified EHR could still be far from having the capability to demonstrate meaningful use. The CMS official also noted that the agency conducted a survey of a sample of providers to learn why they did not continue to participate in the EHR programs and found the following additional reasons:

- some providers did not realize they needed to participate in the program again;
- some providers did not know the deadline for submitting the required information to CMS for the Medicare EHR program, to the states for the Medicaid EHR program, or to both;
- some providers switched EHR vendors and were not ready in time to submit the required information; and
- some providers found it more difficult than anticipated to go from a 90-day reporting period to a full-year reporting period, as required for the second year of participation.

In an effort to reverse this trend, a CMS official told us CMS is working to ensure providers are well-informed regarding program requirements and data submission deadlines. For example, the official told us that CMS is emphasizing requirements and deadlines at meetings with providers, modifying educational materials, and reorganizing the agency's website devoted to the EHR programs.

Program Changes, Including the Increasing Stringency of Requirements and the Implementation of Penalties, Make It Difficult to Estimate Future Participation

Various program changes may affect participation in the EHR programs in the future, making future participation difficult to estimate. Beginning in 2014, Stage 2 requirements for demonstrating meaningful use will be introduced for many providers participating in the EHR programs, requiring providers to demonstrate that they are using their systems in more advanced ways.[56] The increased stringency of these Stage 2 requirements for demonstrating meaningful use may slow participation in the EHR programs. While CMS and ONC have developed guidance materials and trainings to help providers prepare for Stage 2, survey data and statements by organizations representing providers suggest that some providers may be much less capable of demonstrating Stage 2 meaningful use, compared to Stage 1 meaningful use, which might result in reduced participation.[57]

Conversely, other factors may encourage future participation. Penalties for Medicare providers not participating in the Medicare EHR program begin in 2015 and may motivate providers to begin participating in the program or to continue participating in the program.[58] In addition, CMS and ONC have identified certain provider groups as having more difficulty participating in the program and are taking steps to increase participation among these providers. For example, CMS officials told us the agency has partnered with the American Association of Pediatricians to identify states in need of more outreach to encourage pediatricians to participate in the Medicaid EHR program, and ONC's Regional Extension Center program has provided assistance to providers such as professionals in solo practices or rural areas to help them participate in the HER programs.[59] As we previously reported, participation in the Medicare EHR program among rural hospitals and professionals in solo practices increased faster from 2011 to 2012 than participation by hospitals and professionals overall.[60] Furthermore, CMS has made changes to certain program eligibility requirements that may increase the number of providers participating. For example, beginning in 2014, professionals that are hospital-based may receive incentive payments if they can demonstrate that they fund the acquisition, implementation, and maintenance of EHRs in lieu of using a hospital's EHRs.[61] Previously, these professionals were ineligible to participate in the EHR programs.

Providers Exceeded Meaningful Use Requirements for Most Stage 1 Measures, but May Face Challenges with Certain More Stringent Stage 2 Measures

The meaningful use measures reported by providers for 2011 and 2012 indicate that providers used their certified EHR systems more often than required and suggest that many providers who have already reported certain Stage 1 measures will be able to meet most of the more stringent reporting thresholds for similar measures in Stage 2. (See app. IV, table 6.) For 2011 and 2012, Medicare providers that received EHR incentive payments consistently exceeded most meaningful use measure reporting thresholds—that is, a specified percentage of patients or actions required to satisfy the measure—established by CMS and ONC for the EHR programs.[62] Of the 14 hospital meaningful use measures that had thresholds, on average, Medicare hospitals exceeded thresholds by at least 10 percentage points for all measures and by considerably more for many measures. For example, hospitals are required to use computerized provider order entry for more than 30 percent of patients with at least one medication for Stage 1. For both 2011 and 2012, Medicare hospitals reported using computerized provider order entry for medication orders for over 84 percent of patients—about 2.8 times the required threshold for Stage 1. Medicare professionals also greatly exceeded the reporting thresholds.[63] We did not conduct an analysis of meaningful use measures reported by Medicaid providers, but there is some evidence that Medicaid professionals also consistently exceeded required thresholds for 2012.[64] While providers that have not participated in the EHR programs may have different experiences, the fact that Medicare providers and Medicaid professionals that participated in 2011 or 2012—the first two years of Stage 1—generally exceeded most reporting thresholds by wide margins for the measures they reported suggests that they will be able to meet most of the more stringent reporting thresholds in Stage 2.[65] For example, in Stage 2, providers are required to use their certified EHRs to record and chart changes in vital signs for more than 80 percent of patients. Medicare hospitals and professionals exceeded this threshold for both 2011 and 2012, reporting that they met this measure for over 90 percent of patients.

In addition to consistently exceeding most required reporting thresholds, other analyses identify some measures that were frequently reported by providers in Stage 1.[66] (See app. IV, table 7.) For example, close to 100 percent of providers for 2011 and 2012 reported the mandatory Stage 1 measure to record smoking status for patients 13 years and older without claiming allowable exemptions. Certain optional measures, including one related to the electronic exchange of health information, were also frequently reported. For example, over 80 percent of hospitals reported incorporating clinical lab test results into EHRs as structured data.

Although providers were able to report on certain measures that involved the electronic exchange of information, some of the exchange measures may be more challenging for them.[67] Examples of some measures that may be more challenging are the following:

- **Provide summary of care document for each transition of care or referral**. Less than 10 percent of hospitals and less than 15 percent of professionals reported this measure for 2011 and 2012. This measure is optional in Stage 1 and mandatory in Stage 2.
- **Submit public health data**. Fewer than 20 percent of Medicare providers reported the following two public health measures for 2011 and 2012: submit electronic syndromic surveillance data (that is, data collection and analysis to aid identification of outbreaks) to public health agencies and submit electronic data on reportable lab results to public health agencies. Both measures are optional for hospitals in Stage 1 and mandatory for hospitals in Stage 2; the syndromic surveillance measure is optional for professionals in both stages.[68] In addition, these measures become more stringent in Stage 2, requiring ongoing submission of these data rather than just a one-time test of the ability to submit those data, which Stage 1 required.[69]
- **Perform medication reconciliation for patients received from another setting of care or provider of care**. Fewer than 30 percent of Medicare hospitals reported this measure for 2011 and 2012. This measure is optional in Stage 1 and mandatory in Stage 2.

- **Provide patients with their health information electronically**. Less than 35 percent of Medicare hospitals and professionals for both 2011 and 2012 reported the mandatory measure to provide patients with an electronic copy of their health information. Data submitted by the providers that reported this measure indicate that very few patients—often fewer than 4 patients per year for hospitals and 12 patients per year for professionals—requested this electronic information. Additional evidence suggests that this measure was reported by a similar proportion of Medicaid professionals for 2012.[70] In Stage 2, the measure becomes more stringent, by requiring that 5 percent of patients electronically view, download, or transmit their health information to a third party, in addition to requiring hospitals and professionals to provide patients with online access to their health information.

Other information also indicates that providers may face challenges with many of the same exchange-related Stage 2 meaningful use measures identified above. An analysis of the American Hospital Association's 2012 survey of hospitals about technical capabilities related to meaningful use indicates that the least commonly implemented Stage 2 capabilities by acute care hospitals were those related to the electronic exchange of information.[71] Such capabilities included the following: submitting electronic data on reportable lab results to public health agencies; submitting electronic syndromic surveillance data to public health agencies; providing an electronic summary of care document for each transition of care or referral; and providing patients with electronic access to their health information by enabling them to view online, download, and transmit such information. These capabilities are related to optional Stage 1 measures but will be required in Stage 2 or become more complex in Stage 2. An analysis of the National Center for Health Statistics' 2012 National Ambulatory Medical Care Survey shows similar results for physicians. Among the capabilities related to meaningful use measures, office-based physicians were least likely to have routinely submitted electronic data to immunization registries or information systems, or to have routinely communicated with patients using secure messaging. Stage 2 requires professionals to report measures that capture these capabilities, whereas reporting on the first capability was optional in Stage 1 and the second was not a Stage 1 measure.

Consistent with indications from the survey data, stakeholder organizations have also noted concern that providers may have difficulty satisfying certain Stage 2 meaningful use measures due to the changes made to them for Stage 2. Table 4 lists meaningful use measures that organizations identified as challenging—two of which relate to the electronic exchange of information—and includes the requirements for satisfying each measure in Stage 1 and in Stage 2.

Table 4. Changes to Selected Meaningful Use Measures from Stage 1 to Stage 2 of the Electronic Health Record (EHR) Programs

Stage 1	Stage 2
Use computerized provider order entry	
Mandatory measure At least one medication order entered for more than 30 percent of patients with at least one medication	Mandatory measure At least 60 percent of medication orders entered At least 30 percent of laboratory orders entered At least 30 percent of radiology orders entered
Provide patients with their health information electronically	
Mandatory measure[a] Provide electronic copy of health information within 3 days to at least 50 percent of patients who requested an electronic copy • The electronic information can be made available in any form	Mandatory measure[b] Provide electronic access to health information within 36 hours of discharge (hospitals) or 4 days (professionals) to at least 50 percent of patients • Internet-based access is required More than 5 percent of patients view, download, or transmit their health information to a third party
Provide summary care document for each transition of care or referral of care	
Optional measure Provide for more than 50 percent of transitions of care and referrals • Document can be sent electronically or in paper copy • Document must contain the following: diagnostic results, problem list, medication list, medication allergy list, and procedures	Mandatory measure Provide for more than 50 percent of transitions of care and referrals • Document can be sent electronically or in paper copy • Document must contain the following: patient name; referringor transitioning provider's name and office contact information (professionals only);

Stage 1	Stage 2
	procedures; encounter diagnosis; immunizations; laboratory test results; vital signs (height, weight, blood pressure, body mass index); smoking status; functional status; demographic information (preferred language, sex, race, ethnicity, date of birth); care plan field; care team; reason for referral (professional only); discharge instructions (hospital only); current problem list; current medication list; and current medication allergy list Electronically transmit document for more than 10 percent of transitions of care and referrals Conduct one or more tests of successful electronic exchange of document with either a provider with a different certified EHR vendor or the CMS-designated test EHR

Source: GAO analysis of Office of the National Coordinator for Health Information Technology (ONC) regulations and CMS guidance.

Note: The following provider organizations identified these meaningful use measures as being challenging in Stage 2: the American Hospital Association, the American Medical Association, and the College of Healthcare Information Management Executives.

[a]This was the Stage 1 requirement for 2011 through 2013. Beginning in 2014 the Stage 1 requirement is to provide electronic internet-based access to health information within 36 hours of discharge (hospitals) or 4 days (professionals) to at least 50 percent of patients.

[b]CMS guidance notes that the Stage 2 version of this measure replaces the following Stage 1 measure that was required for hospitals: "provide patients with electronic copy of discharge instructions at the time of discharge" for more than 50 percent of patients who requested that information within 3 business days and the Stage 1 measure that was optional for professionals:

> "provide patients with timely electronic access to their health information" to at least 10 percent of patients within 4 business days.

A CMS official noted that although providers have expressed concern about their ability to meet the Stage 2 requirements, similar concerns existed prior to Stage 1 regarding the thresholds established for certain measures and the data suggest that providers have exceeded thresholds established by CMS for the Stage 1 requirements. This official also explained efforts to help providers to prepare to satisfy the Stage 2 meaningful use measures. CMS has been modifying its materials and holding training sessions and discussions with various provider groups. In anticipation of obstacles to the exchange of health information and in order to accelerate electronic exchange even among providers not eligible for incentive payments from the EHR programs, ONC and CMS issued a request for information in March 2013 to, among other things, solicit feedback on the challenges to the electronic exchange of health information and on possible mechanisms to overcome those challenges.[72] Using the information collected, CMS and ONC issued a strategy in August 2013 for how they expect to advance health information exchange, which includes various steps the agencies plan to take under three broad categories—accelerating health information exchange, advancing standards and interoperability, and patient engagement.[73] Ongoing work is examining the key challenges to the electronic exchange of health information that have been reported by providers and stakeholders and HHS's efforts to address those challenges.

HHS Lacks a Comprehensive Strategy to Help Ensure Reliability of EHR Data Collected to Improve Quality of Care

The lack of a comprehensive strategy limits HHS's ability to ensure that the department can reliably use the CQMs collected in certified EHRs for quality measurement activities. According to internal control standards, an agency must have relevant and reliable information to help it achieve its mission and goals. In order to drive quality improvement and accountability and to effectively utilize CQM data collected in EHRs for HHS's quality measurement activities, the data collected must be reliable, that is, both accurate and complete. Data that are not reliable limit the credibility of the information and may present a risk to individuals or entities making decisions based on the data, such as to a patient choosing a hospital for treatment, or to CMS when applying a payment modifier resulting in an increase or reduction to a physician's reimbursement.

CMS and ONC have made changes to the specifications, certification criteria, and certification program to address some of the reliability concerns with the CQMs that providers were generally required to collect and report from 2011 to 2013 to demonstrate meaningful use (that is, using 2011-edition EHRs). These changes are incorporated into EHRs that will be used by participating providers in all stages of meaningful use from 2014 to 2016 (that is, 2014-edition EHRs). The changes made as a result of the concerns identified include the following.

Specifications

CMS made changes to CQM specifications—that is, the documentation that describes to providers, technology developers, and others how data on CQMs were to be collected through EHRs. These changes were made to correct previously identified errors and to help ensure the feasibility of implementing CQMs in the electronic format—that is, to ensure that the required data are readily available or can be collected in EHRs without undue burden. Problems with feasibility can compromise the accuracy or completeness of the data.[74]

Certification Criteria

To address providers' concern that their 2011- edition EHRs did not collect all of the data elements necessary to calculate the CQMs, ONC modified the CQM-related certification criteria.

Specifically, 2014-edition EHRs must collect each of the data elements associated with a specific CQM to be certified for that measure.[75]

Certification Program

The program for certifying 2011-edition EHRs did not test whether the EHR system correctly collected and calculated the CQMs. However, beginning with the certification of 2014-edition EHRs, the certification bodies and testing laboratories will test whether EHRs accurately collect and calculate CQMs. These tests will be performed using a certification testing tool developed by ONC, known as Cypress.[76] Further, beginning in 2014, the certification bodies will be required by ONC to conduct specific annual surveillance activities to determine whether 2014-edition EHRs are functioning as intended after being implemented by providers. CQMs have been identified as a priority area for these surveillance activities, which may help to inform CMS and ONC on whether the changes they have made to the specifications, certification criteria, and certification program are improving the reliability of CQMs, as intended, and whether further changes are needed.

CMS and ONC officials indicated the changes made thus far should help to address reliability concerns, but provider experience with 2014-edition EHRs will be an important gauge of the effectiveness of the changes. 77 Furthermore, there are still issues that could result in reliability problems, hindering CMS's ability to use the data for its quality measurement activities. For example, after EHRs are certified as 2014-edition EHRs, the agencies do not require them to be recertified following updates to the specifications, which may be made annually or more frequently, or following updates to the certification testing tool.[78] Thus, different providers may report CQMs based on and tested to different requirements. CMS has taken some steps to mitigate the potential effect of these issues on the reliability of CQM data submitted by professionals who electronically submit CQM data by requiring them to report CQMs collected using EHR technology based on and tested to the most recent version of the electronic specifications. However, this variability may limit the ability to reliably compare quality across other providers, including hospitals, and undermines efforts CMS officials said they are taking to ensure that the CQMs lead to standardized, consistent data reporting. Another issue that may affect reliability is that many providers reported at least one CQM based on few patients, which may result in data that are not statistically reliable and therefore should not be used in quality measurement.[79] We analyzed data submitted by providers to demonstrate meaningful use under the Medicare EHR program for 2011 and 2012 and found that 90 percent of hospitals and 50 percent of professionals reported at least one CQM based on few patients for 2012, a slight increase compared to 2011, when 86 percent of hospitals and 46 percent of professionals reported at least one CQM based on few patients.[80]

In addition, stakeholder organizations continue to have concerns about reliability. CHIME members indicated that they do not think the specifications required to generate CQMs using 2014-edition EHRs will substantially improve the reliability of the data collected in Stage 2. They noted that the collection of CQM data includes data elements not currently captured by EHRs, and the data elements are not automatically part of most clinicians' workflow (that is, incorporated into the tasks performed during the delivery of routine care). Due to these obstacles, CHIME members are concerned that clinicians will not consistently collect the required data elements, ultimately leading to problems with CQM reliability and comparability. CMS and ONC are making changes to the process used to develop new measures, which includes greater consideration of clinician workflow and provider burden. However, new CQMs will not be available until the beginning of Stage 3 in 2017.

Another concern expressed by stakeholder organizations such as the American Health Information Management Association, the American Hospital Association, the American Medical Association, the Healthcare Information and Management Systems Society, and The Joint Commission is that the CQMs generated from EHRs—which are based on electronically specified measures and are extracted automatically from EHRs—do not produce results that are comparable to corresponding measures based on data obtained through other methods, such as through manual abstraction of patient medical records by trained professionals. In its fiscal year 2014 Inpatient Prospective Payment System final rule, CMS noted that it intends to use the electronic CQM data submitted voluntarily by hospitals to assess the differences in performance rates from CQMs collected using EHRs and CQMs collected through chart-abstraction.[81] However, CMS did not indicate when this study would be completed or describe how it would be designed. Designing the study to control for any other systematic differences between providers that use EHRs and other providers could have an important effect on CMS's ability to understand the extent and implications of potential differences in performance rates.

Although CMS officials told us that they were beginning to develop an approach to validate CQM data generated from EHRs, HHS has not yet developed a comprehensive strategy to address concerns with the reliability of CQMs collected using certified EHRs. Consistent with GPRAMA and our prior work, which identifies several important practices that can guide agencies in planning and implementing an effective government program, a comprehensive strategy would establish objectives, steps to achieve results, priorities, and milestones and identify the steps necessary to achieve desired results. Addressing the concerns is important to ensure that the CQM data can be reliably used for CMS's quality measurement activities as well as providers' quality improvement activities. For example, CMS plans to use CQMs collected and submitted via EHRs by certain professionals in 2014 to determine which providers will be subject to payment modifications under the Value Based Payment Modifier program in 2016. For hospitals, CMS officials told us that as part of their approach to validating data, they plan to use electronically submitted CQMs to develop monitoring processes to help inform them about the consistency and reliability of the data reported. Also for hospitals, CMS officials told us that they expect to introduce a process that is as robust as the one that is currently used for the IQR program under which a CMS contractor conducts an independent analysis to verify that the data submitted accurately reflect the information in the medical record.[82] CMS officials told us that the agency's plans for validating CQM data are preliminary, but the agency has stated that it intends to develop and propose a strategy for hospital data in 2014 as part of the agency's annual rulemaking process. While the IQR program may provide a model for validating data collected by hospitals using certified EHRs, no comparable model or process exists that could be considered when developing a validation strategy for data collected by professionals using certified EHRs. Until HHS establishes and implements a comprehensive strategy to ensure the reliability of CQMs collected using certified EHRs, it will be unclear whether the department's plans are sufficient to address the concerns, and therefore it will be uncertain when the CQM data can be reliably used to help assess provider performance, improve quality, and adjust provider payments.

HHS, CMS, and ONC have established some performance measures for the EHR programs that are tied to strategic goals, but have not established performance measures for the goals most relevant to the intended outcomes of the EHR programs—that is, goals related to improving health care quality, efficiency, and patient safety. Establishing performance measures tied to goals is important for ensuring that agencies' activities move them closer to accomplishing these goals, according to our guidance to federal agencies on effectively implementing GPRAMA, which describes leading practices for how federal agencies should assess their performance.[83] Our guidance also notes that agencies should use information that performance measures provide to improve processes and set improvement goals. However, as the agencies have not established performance measures to assess outcomes, they are therefore unable to use the information such measures would provide.

Performance Measures for the EHR Programs Do Not Assess Outcomes Such As Improved Quality, Efficiency, and Patient Safety

Based on review of relevant documents, we identified two categories of department and agency goals that are particularly relevant to the EHR programs—(1) adoption and meaningful use of EHRs, which is focused on program processes; and (2) improving quality, efficiency, and patient safety, which is focused on program outcomes. For the first category, HHS, CMS, and ONC have established 26 performance measures that allow them to track program processes, such as provider participation levels.[84] The majority of these measures focus on participation in the EHR programs as measured by meeting requirements for adoption and meaningful use of EHRs. For example, HHS, CMS, and ONC have performance measures for the number of eligible providers who receive an incentive payment from the EHR programs for the successful adoption or meaningful use of EHRs. ONC has also recently established performance measures related to exchanging information electronically, in keeping with the emphasis on the electronic exchange of information in Stage 2. For example, ONC has established a performance measure for the percentage of nonfederal acute care hospitals that are electronically sharing summary of care records with providers outside their organization. (See app. V, table 8 for a list of the department- and agency-level strategic goals and 26 associated performance measures for this category.)

For these established performance measures, the agencies have developed corresponding performance targets and track results against those targets. For example, ONC has set a fiscal year 2014 target that 65 percent of nonfederal acute hospitals electronically share summary of care records with providers outside of their organization. These performance targets are publicly released alongside the performance measures and actual results in the annual ONC and CMS budget justifications and the HHS online performance appendix.[85] The agencies told us they use this performance information to set the broader strategic direction for the agency and may also use the information to make changes to the programs to improve performance.

However, although HHS, CMS, and ONC have established important performance measures for the goals related to adoption and meaningful use of EHRs, they have not established measures linked to the second category of goals, which would help them to track program outcomes such as health care quality, efficiency, and patient safety. (See app. V, table 9 for a list of the department- and agency-level strategic goals for this category.) Outcome measures would enable the agencies to measure whether the EHR programs' intended effects are being achieved, rather than just the number of providers that satisfied the requirements necessary to demonstrate meaningful use. ONC's strategic plan states that the meaningful use of EHRs—which, as explained above, the agencies track using several performance measures—is a necessary step to improve health care quality, efficiency, and patient safety.

However, meaningful use is not sufficient to achieve these outcomes on its own. The plan notes that the EHR programs are an HIT investment made in lockstep with various other reform efforts such as patient-centered medical homes and that EHRs will contribute to improvements in health care quality, efficiency, and patient safety when used in support of these other reform efforts. Therefore, outcome measures—and the subsequent use of the information they provide—could be beneficial to evaluating how the EHR programs interact with other reform efforts. Furthermore, ONC has acknowledged the need to develop performance measures to track patient safety, in part due to concerns that EHRs could have some unintended consequences that cause patient harm. However, ONC has not yet developed these potential measures.[86]

Without performance measures linked to the goals of improved health care quality, efficiency, and patient safety, CMS and ONC are limited in their abilities to determine the effectiveness of the EHR programs in improving outcomes. CMS and ONC may lack critical information necessary to establish program priorities and subsequently make program adjustments based on progress toward these outcomes. CMS and ONC officials have indicated that they do not expect to observe progress toward achieving the intended outcomes of improved health care quality, efficiency, and patient safety until at least Stage 3 of the EHR programs, which is not expected until 2017. However, establishing outcome-oriented performance measures before results are expected is a valuable practice to ensure that the agencies can make program adjustments as needed and are prepared to monitor outcomes and to establish baseline values, which can be useful for developing performance targets and assessing progress toward goals. Moreover, consistent with our guidance, outcome measures could be useful to guide the development and prioritization of Stage 3 requirements, which the agencies anticipate undertaking in 2014.

While the agencies have not established outcome-related performance measures, agency officials told us they are conducting some evaluations to assess the effect of the EHR programs on outcomes. For example, ONC officials told us that CMS, ONC, and the Agency for Healthcare Research and Quality were working on a study to assess the effect of electronic prescribing on quality and efficiency using Medicare Part D claims, specifically, to determine whether electronic prescribing for diabetes patients is associated with a reduced risk of adverse drug events.[87] (See app. VI for a summary of program evaluations assessing the EHR programs' effects on outcomes.) However, these program evaluations—in contrast to performance measures—

capture only a specific period of time, and, as a result, do not allow for ongoing monitoring of the EHR programs' effectiveness.

CONCLUSION

The EHR programs were intended to be long-term solutions—with multiple stages implemented over several years—to help address longstanding, significant barriers to greater use of EHRs as tools for improving outcomes such as health care quality, efficiency, and patient safety. The first stage of the EHR programs, from 2011 to 2012, has shown sizeable increases in the number of providers who have adopted and meaningfully used EHRs. This early measure of implementation still leaves substantial room to further increase meaningful use among certain providers. Implementation of the subsequent stages, which will increasingly emphasize the use of more advanced features of EHRs, will place more demands on providers through more stringent requirements, but could also increase the potential for achieving better outcomes. Because of the programs' design to evolve over multiple years and stages, HHS has opportunities to make adjustments and closely monitor the programs to ensure that they remain on track to achieve their intended results.

One key feature of EHRs that shows a need for adjustment relates to the CQMs. We describe several issues regarding the reliability of CQM data—for example, providers may be reporting CQMs based on and tested to different specifications. The reliability of CQM data collected using certified EHRs is especially important due to the potential risk of making decisions—such as paying providers for performance—based on unreliable CQM data. CMS and ONC lack a comprehensive strategy that would allow them to ensure the reliability of CQM data collected using EHRs, in accordance with the internal control standard requiring an agency to have relevant and reliable information to achieve its mission and goals. Without a comprehensive strategy, the agencies may be limited in their abilities to reliably compare quality across providers or use CQM data collected through EHRs for a variety of quality measurement and pay-for-performance activities, thus restricting efforts to improve quality and efficiency.

Another area that merits attention relates to HHS's ability to ensure that the EHR programs are on track to meet their goals. While the EHR programs are ultimately intended to improve outcomes such as health care quality, efficiency, and patient safety, the agencies have not established performance measures for monitoring progress toward achieving these improvements. Although HHS expects that EHRs can help achieve improved outcomes as well as support various other health care reform efforts that are also intended to improve care, that result is not yet assured. As established by our guidance to federal agencies, monitoring progress toward specific outcomes could allow HHS to make adjustments to the EHR programs throughout their implementation, such as adjusting priorities or requirements. Without such monitoring, the agencies will not be well positioned to understand how challenges affecting key parts of the programs, such as ensuring the reliability of CQM data or increasing providers' abilities to exchange health information, might be affecting the programs' overall ability to achieve their goals, reducing HHS's ability to make course corrections.

Recommendations for Executive Action

To more effectively use CQMs to assess provider performance, the Secretary of Health and Human Services should direct CMS and ONC to take the following action:

- Develop a comprehensive strategy for ensuring that CQM data collected and reported using certified EHR technology are reliable, including testing for and mitigation of reliability issues arising from variance in certified EHR systems tested to different CQM specifications.

To ensure that CMS and ONC can effectively monitor the effect of the EHR programs and progress made toward goals, the Secretary of Health and Human Services should direct the agencies to take the following two actions:

- Develop performance measures to assess outcomes of the EHR programs—including any effects on health care quality, efficiency, and patient safety and other health care reform efforts that are intended to work toward similar outcomes—and
- Use the information these performance measures provide to make program adjustments, as appropriate, to better achieve program goals.

Agency Comments and Our Evaluation

HHS provided written comments on a draft of this report and one technical comment. HHS agreed that data reliability and performance monitoring are important, but neither agreed nor disagreed with our recommendations. Regarding our first recommendation, HHS stated that the reliability and validity of CQM data are of paramount importance. HHS also stated that ONC and CMS work together to continually refine strategies to improve the reliability and efficiency of collecting, analyzing, and sharing CQM data collected using certified EHR technology. HHS did not, however, identify any specific actions the agencies might take to improve CQM reliability or whether those actions would include developing a comprehensive strategy. HHS also noted the importance of the certification testing tool, known as Cypress, which it stated ensures the reliability of CQM data collected using 2014-edition EHRs. While the addition of testing to ensure that 2014-edition EHRs accurately collect and calculate CQMs is an improvement over the process used to certify 2011-edition EHRs—during which such tests were not conducted—our report raises other reliability issues that would not be addressed by the certification testing tool alone. Regarding our second and third recommendations, HHS agreed that outcome-oriented performance measures that link participation in the EHR programs with discrete improvements in health care quality, efficiency, and safety would be useful for evaluating the extent to which improvements are achieved. HHS also noted that ONC oversees evaluation activities that have provided interim program results and conducts policy research and analytic projects that will enable the development of outcome-oriented performance measures. However, HHS did not provide any details on the timing or content of outcome-oriented performance measures that CMS and ONC might develop.

Linda T. Kohn
Director, Health Care

Appendix I: Effect of the HITECH Act on Health Insurance Premiums

The Health Information Technology for Economic and Clinical Health (HITECH) Act mandates us to report on, among other things, the impact of the

HITECH Act on health insurance premiums. In 2009, the Congressional Budget Office stated an expectation that nationwide adoption of health information technology such as electronic health records (EHR) would reduce total spending on health care and predicted that lower health care costs for private payers would result in lower health insurance premiums in the private sector.

To describe the effect of the HITECH Act on health insurance premiums, we contacted representatives from America's Health Insurance Plans, the American Academy of Actuaries, the Blue Cross Blue Shield Association, and four health insurance companies.[1] None of the seven organizations we spoke to had done any research to look at the impact of the HITECH Act on health insurance premiums. Three organizations also indicated that the HITECH Act's effect on health insurance premiums would be difficult to isolate from the various other drivers of health insurance premium costs. For example, one organization noted that the health insurance industry is also in the midst of implementing the Patient Protection and Affordable Care Act, suggesting the reforms arising from that legislation are also affecting health insurance premium costs.

Five of the seven organizations offered anecdotes or speculation as to the potential effect of the HITECH Act—and particularly the adoption and meaningful use of EHRs as encouraged by the EHR programs—on health insurance premiums. One organization told us that there is evidence that widely implemented payment and delivery reform—particularly the patient-centered medical home, of which EHRs are an important element—has led to reductions in health care utilization and, in some cases, generated savings, which may eventually affect health insurance premiums. Another organization said that implementing the HITECH Act and the Patient Protection and Affordable Care Act has increased administrative costs and expressed concern that if the organization's administrative costs increase due to changes in requirements, they may rise above the 15 to 20 percent level allowed under medical loss ratio requirements.[2]

APPENDIX II: SCOPE AND METHODOLOGY

This appendix provides additional details regarding our analysis of (1) participation in the Medicare and Medicaid Electronic Health Record (EHR) programs; (2) meaningful use measures and clinical quality measures (CQM) Medicare providers reported to the Centers for Medicare & Medicaid Services

(CMS) to demonstrate meaningful use; and (3) 2012 survey data collected by the National Center for Health Statistics.

To ensure the reliability of the data, we interviewed officials from CMS, reviewed relevant documentation, and conducted electronic testing to identify missing data and obvious errors. On the basis of these activities, we determined that the data were sufficiently reliable for our analysis.

Analysis of Participation in the Medicare and Medicaid EHR Programs

We conducted several analyses to report on participation in the Medicare and Medicaid EHR programs for the 2011 and 2012 program years.[1] Specifically, we analyzed data that CMS collected in the National Level Repository through October 23, 2013. As a result, we generally included full-year information for both years in our analysis of the Medicare EHR program.[2] However, our analysis does not contain complete information for the Medicaid EHR program for the 2012 program year because, according to CMS, 14 states and the District of Columbia had not yet completed their determinations of which hospitals and professionals had met all the requirements to receive incentive payments for 2012. We used these data to conduct the following analyses.

- We estimated the percentage of eligible providers awarded an incentive payment from either the Medicare or the Medicaid EHR program. We determined the number of providers that were awarded a Medicare or Medicaid (or, in the case of some hospitals, both) EHR incentive payment by counting the number of providers that had an incentive payment disbursed to them for 2011 and for 2012[3] We divided the number of providers awarded incentive payments from either program by the total number of eligible providers CMS estimated in its Stage 1 final rule.[4] Specifically, CMS estimated that 5,013 hospitals and 521,600 professionals were eligible for the Medicare or Medicaid EHR program for 2011 and 5,013 hospitals and 527,200 professionals for 2012.
- We determined the total amount of Medicare and Medicaid EHR incentive payments awarded to providers each year by summing the Medicare and Medicaid EHR incentive payments awarded to providers for each program year.[5]

- We estimated the percentage of providers that were awarded a Medicare or Medicaid (or, in the case of some hospitals, both) EHR incentive payment for 2011 but not for 2012 by determining the number of providers that had a Medicare or Medicaid EHR incentive payment disbursed to them for 2011 but not for 2012.[6] For the Medicaid EHR program, we limited this analysis to providers that were awarded incentive payments from 36 states that, according to CMS, had completed their determinations of which providers would receive incentive payments for the 2011 and 2012 Medicaid EHR program years as of October 23, 2013.

Analysis of Meaningful Use Measures and CQMs Medicare Providers Reported to CMS to Demonstrate Meaningful Use

We conducted several analyses of meaningful use measures and CQMs providers reported to CMS to demonstrate meaningful use under the Medicare EHR program for 2011 and 2012. We analyzed data that CMS collected in the National Level Repository through October 23, 2013. We did not analyze meaningful use measure or CQM data submitted by hospitals or professionals who received incentive payments from the Medicare Advantage EHR program or CQM data submitted by providers to one of the electronic reporting pilots that were available for the 2012 program year.[7] For each of the following analyses, we compared reporting by program year.

- We determined the extent to which providers exceeded the reporting thresholds CMS established for a subset of the meaningful use measures (14 hospital measures and 16 professional measures) by determining providers' average reporting rate for each applicable measure and comparing this rate to the threshold CMS established for the measures.
- We determined the frequency with which providers reported meaningful use measures without claiming exemptions, by calculating the percentage of providers that reported meaningful use measures but excluding from the calculation those providers that reported to CMS that a measure was not relevant to them. A provider may claim exemptions from reporting some measures if the provider meets certain criteria specific to the individual measures. For example, the measure may not be relevant to the provider's patient populations or

clinical practices, the provider may have conducted too few actions to be measured, or the provider may not have been able to perform the action. The agency allows providers to claim exemptions from reporting certain meaningful use measures to help ensure that providers with all types of patient populations and clinical practices could potentially demonstrate meaningful use. For 2011 and 2012, hospitals were permitted to claim exemptions from reporting 7 meaningful use measures and professionals from reporting 14 meaningful use measures.[8]

- We determined the extent to which providers had few patients who could be included in the calculation of at least one CQM.[9] CQMs that capture a small number of patients may be unreliable measures of quality because relatively small changes in the number of patients who experienced the care processes or outcomes targeted by the measure can generate large shifts in the calculated percentage for the measure. CMS has recognized in other programs that including a small number of patients in the calculation of a CQM is a reliability issue. For example, on the agency's Hospital Compare website, which publicly reports CQMs by hospital, CMS indicates whether the number of patients included in a particular measure calculation was based on fewer than 25 patients and was thus too small to reliably tell how well the hospital was performing. For our analysis, we identified CQMs as unreliable if fewer than 7 patients met inclusion criteria for the calculation the provider reported for a 90-day reporting period—that is, during the provider's first year demonstrating meaningful use. For providers whose second year demonstrating meaningful use was 2012, the reporting period is a full year. Therefore, for these providers we identified CQMs as unreliable if fewer than 25 patients met the inclusion criteria for the calculation.

Analysis of 2012 survey data collected by the National Center for Health Statistics

We analyzed output of the National Ambulatory Medical Care Survey, an annual, nationally representative survey of office-based physicians conducted by the National Center for Health Statistics in the Centers for Disease Control and Prevention. The survey captures information about computerized capabilities of office-based physicians' EHRs—which are related to meaningful use measures— including whether those capabilities are routinely used. We analyzed output from the 2012 survey obtained from the National Center for Health Statistics. We limited our analysis to office-based physicians who reported using an EHR or an electronic medical record system and who reported having patient care revenue from Medicare or Medicaid (69.0 percent of weighted responses). We then identified the computerized capabilities that were least likely to have been routinely used and determined, using a crosswalk of meaningful use measures and survey responses available from the Office of the National Coordinator for Health Information Technology (ONC), whether those capabilities were comparable to Stage 2 meaningful use measures.[10] We also determined whether the computerized capabilities that were least likely to have been routinely used were related to electronic health information, based on information obtained from CMS and ONC.

APPENDIX III: STAGE 1 AND STAGE 2 MEANINGFUL USE MEASURES

In general, to receive incentive payments from the Medicare or Medicaid Electronic Health Record (EHR) programs in Stage 1 or Stage 2, hospitals must report on a total of 19, and professionals must report on a total of 20, measures regarding their use of certified EHR technology, known as meaningful use measures.[1] For certain meaningful use measures, a provider may report to the Centers for Medicare & Medicaid Services (CMS) that the measures are not relevant if the provider meets certain criteria specific to the individual measures; this is referred to as claiming an exemption. For example, the measure may not be relevant to the provider's patient population or clinical practice, the provider may have conducted too few actions to be measured, or the provider may not have been able to perform the action. Table 5 lists the meaningful use measures for each stage and provider type and identifies whether the measure was mandatory or optional and whether it was identified by the Office of the National Coordinator for Health Information Technology (ONC) and CMS as being related to the electronic exchange of health information.

Table 5. Meaningful Use Measures for Professionals and Hospitals, Stages 1 and 2 of the Electronic Health Record (EHR) Programs

		Mandatory (●) or optional (o) measure			
		Hospitals		Professionals	
Meaningful use measure	Exchange - related	Stage 1	Stage 2	Stage 1	Stage 2
Use computerized provider order entry: For Stage 1: Use for at least one medication order for more than 30 percent of patients with at least one medication in their medication lists; for Stage 2, use for more than 60 percent of medication orders, 30 percent of laboratory orders, and 30 percent of radiology orders		●	●	●[a]	●[a]
Implement drug-drug and drug-allergy interaction checks: Enable the EHR system's ability to check for these interactions		●	[b]	●	[b]
Maintain an up-to-date problem list of current and active diagnoses: Record list of current and active diagnoses or indicate no known problems for more than 80 percent of patients		●	[c]	●	[c]
Generate and transmit permissible prescriptions electronically: For hospitals for Stage 2, generate, transmit, and check each prescription for the existence of a relevant drug formulary for more than 10 percent of hospital discharge prescriptions; for professionals, generate and transmit more than 40 percent (for Stage 1) or more than 50 percent (for Stage 2) of permissible prescriptions electronically and for Stage 2 also check each prescription for the existence of a relevant formulary	Yes		O[a]	●[a]	●[a]
Maintain active medication list: Record at least one entry or indicate no current prescriptions for more than 80 percent of patients		●	[c]	●	[c]

Table 5. (Continued)

		Mandatory (•) or optional (o) measure			
		Hospitals		Professionals	
Meaningful use measure	Exchange - related	Stage 1	Stage 2	Stage 1	Stage 2
Maintain active medication allergy list: Record at least one entry or indicate no known medication allergies for more than 80 percent of patients		•	[c]	•	[c]
Record demographics: Record preferred language, sex, race, ethnicity, and date of birth for more than 50 percent (for Stage 1) or more than 80 percent (for Stage 2) of patients; hospitals must also record date and preliminary cause of death in the event of mortality		•	•	•	•
Record and chart changes in vital signs: For Stage 1, record height, weight, and blood pressure for more than 50 percent of patients age 2 and older. For Stage 2, for more than 80 percent of all patients, record blood pressure (for patients age 3 and older) and/or height and weight. For both stages, calculate and display body mass index and plot and display growth charts for children age 2 through 20 (for Stage 1) or patients age 0 through 20 (for Stage 2)		•	•	•[a]	•[a]
Record smoking status for patients 13 years old or older: Record smoking status for more than 50 percent (for Stage 1) or more than 80 percent (for Stage 2) of patients age 13 and older		•[a]	•[a]	•[a]	•[a]
Report clinical quality measures to CMS		•	[d]	•	[d]

		Mandatory (•) or optional (o) measure			
		Hospitals		Professionals	
Meaningful use measure	Exchange - related	Stage 1	Stage 2	Stage 1	Stage 2
Implement clinical decision support: For Stage 1: implement one clinical decision support rule related to specialty or high clinical priority along with the ability to track compliance with that rule. For Stage 2: Implement five clinical decision support interventions related to four or more clinical quality measures or to high-priority health conditions; for hospitals, it is suggested that one of the five interventions be related to improving efficiency. For Stage 2, enable and implement drug-drug and drug-allergy interaction checks		•	•	•	•[a]
Provide patients with their health information electronically: For Stage 1: provide information (for hospitals and professionals, provide diagnostic test results, problem list, medication lists, and medication allergies, and for hospitals also provide discharge summary and procedures) within 3 business days to more than 50 percent of patients who requested to receive that information electronically. For Stage 2: Provide more than 50 percent of patients with online access to their health information within 36 hours of discharge (for hospitals) or 4 days (for professionals); more than 5 percent of patients view, download, or transmit their health information to a third party.	Yes	•[a, e]	•[a]	•[a, e]	•[a]
For hospitals, provide patients with electronic copy of discharge instructions at the time of discharge, upon request; for professionals, provide patients with clinical summaries for each office visit: For hospitals,	Yes	•[a]	[f]	•[a, g]	•[a]

Table 5. (Continued)

		Mandatory (●) or optional (o) measure			
		Hospitals		Professionals	
Meaningful use measure	Exchange - related	Stage 1	Stage 2	Stage 1	Stage 2
provide information for more than 50 percent of patients who requested that information; for professionals, provide information for more than 50 percent of visits within 3 business days for Stage 1 or 1 business day for Stage 2					
Exchange key clinical information electronically: Perform at least one test of EHR technology's capacity to exchange key clinical information	Yes	●[h]		●[h]	
Protect electronic health information created or maintained by the certified EHR technology: Conduct or review a security risk analysis (for Stage 1 and Stage 2) including addressing encryption/security of data stored in certified EHR technology (for Stage 2 only), implement security updates as necessary, and correct identified security deficiencies		●	●	●	●
Implement drug formulary checks: Enable this functionality and maintain access to at least one internal or external formulary		○	[i]	○[a]	[i]
Incorporate clinical lab test results into EHR as structured data: Incorporate into the EHR technology more than 40 percent (for Stage 1) or 55 percent (for Stage 2) of the clinical lab test results ordered whose results are positive, negative, or in numerical format	Yes	○[j]	●[j]	○[a, j]	●[a,j]
Generate patient lists by specific conditions: Generate at least one report listing patients with a specific condition to use for quality improvement, reduction of disparities, research, or outreach		○	●	○	●

		Mandatory (●) or optional (o) measure			
		Hospitals		Professionals	
Meaningful use measure	Exchange - related	Stage 1	Stage 2	Stage 1	Stage 2
Send patient reminders per patient preference for preventive or follow-up care: For Stage 1: send appropriate reminders to more than 20 percent of patients age 65 and older or age 5 and younger; For Stage 2: identify patients who should receive reminders and send reminders to more than 10 percent of patients who have had two or more office visits within 24 months before the reporting period				○[a]	●[a]
Identify patient-specific education resources and provide those resources to the patient if appropriate: Provide to more than 10 percent of patients		○	●	○	●[a]
Perform medication reconciliation for patients received from another setting of care or provider of care: Perform for more than 50 percent of transitions of care	Yes	○[g]	●[g]	○[a, g]	●[a,g]
Provide summary of care document for each transition of care or referral: For Stage 1 and Stage 2, provide for more than 50 percent of transitions of care and referrals; for Stage 2 also (a) provide for more than 10 percent of transitions of care and referrals either electronically transmitted using certified EHR technology or through an exchange with a Nationwide Health Information Network Exchange participant or in a way that is consistent with the Nationwide Health Information Network (b) conduct one or more successful electronic exchanges of a summary of care document with a recipient with EHR technology designed by a different developer than the sender's or conduct one or more successful tests with the CMS-designated test EHR	Yes	○	●	○[a]	●[a]

Table 5. (Continued)

		Mandatory (•) or optional (o) measure			
		Hospitals		Professionals	
Meaningful use measure	Exchange - related	Stage 1	Stage 2	Stage 1	Stage 2
Submit electronic data to immunization registries or immunization information systems: For Stage 1, perform at least one test of EHR technology's capacity to submit data to immunization registries and, if test is successful, institute regular reporting; for Stage 2, demonstrate successful ongoing submission of data to immunization registries	Yes	O[a]	•[a]	O[a]	•[a]
Submit electronic syndromic surveillance data to public health agencies: For Stage 1, perform at least one test of EHR technology's capacity to submit data to public health agencies and, if test is successful, institute regular reporting; for Stage 2, demonstrate successful ongoing submission of data to public health agencies	Yes	O[a]	•[a]	O[a]	O[a]
Submit electronic data on reportable lab results to public health agencies: For stage 1, perform at least one test of EHR technology's capacity to submit data (as required by state or local law) to public health agencies and, if test is successful, institute regular reporting; for Stage 2, demonstrate successful ongoing submission of data (as required by state or local law) to public health agencies	Yes	O[a]	•[a]		
Record advance directives for patients 65 years or older: Record indication of advance directive status for more than 50 percent of all unique patients age 65 and older		O[a]	O[a]		

		Mandatory (•) or optional (o) measure			
		Hospitals		Professionals	
Meaningful use measure	Exchange - related	Stage 1	Stage 2	Stage 1	Stage 2
Use secure electronic messaging to communicate with patients: More than 5 percent of patients sent the professional a secure message	Yes				•[a]
Provide patients with timely electronic access to their health information: Provide electronic access to health information (including lab results, problem list, medication lists, and allergies) to at least 10 percent of patients within 4 business days	Yes			o[a, k]	[f]
Automatically track medications using assistive technologies and an electronic medication administration record: Track all doses using electronic medication administration record for more than 10 percent of medication orders			•[a]		
Record electronic notes in patient records: Enter at least one electronic progress note that is text searchable for more than 30 percent of patients during the reporting period			o		o
Ensure that imaging results and accompanying information are accessible through certified EHR technology: Make more than 10 percent of all tests with one or more images accessible through certified EHR technology	Yes		o		o[a]
Record patient family health history as structured data: Record family health history for one or more first-degree relatives for more than 20 percent of patients			o		o[a]
Demonstrate capability to identify and report cancer cases to public health central cancer registry: Demonstrate successful ongoing submission of cancer case information from certified EHR technology to a public health central cancer registry	Yes				o[a]

Table 5. (Continued)

		Mandatory (•) or optional (o) measure			
		Hospitals		Professionals	
Meaningful use measure	Exchange - related	Stage 1	Stage 2	Stage 1	Stage 2
Demonstrate capability to identify and report specific cases to a specialized registry: Demonstrate successful ongoing submission of specific case information from certified EHR technology to a specialized registry other than a cancer registry	Yes				O[a]
Provide structured electronic lab results to ambulatory providers: Send structured electronic clinical lab results to the ordering provider for more than 20 percent of electronic lab orders	Yes		O		

Source: GAO analysis of CMS guidance and of information obtained from CMS and ONC officials.

Notes: Mandatory meaningful use measures are designated as (•) and optional meaningful use measures (the set of measures from which CMS allows providers the flexibility to select a subset of measures to report) as (O). The "exchange-related" column identifies meaningful use measures that are related to electronic health information exchange according to CMS, ONC, or both agencies. In the Medicare and Medicaid EHR programs, professionals include doctors of medicine and dental surgery. In the Medicaid EHR program, professionals also include nurse practitioners, certified nurse-midwives, and certain physician assistants.

[a]Providers may claim exemptions from reporting the measure if they meet certain criteria specific to the measure.

[b]For Stage 2, this measure was incorporated into the "implement clinical decision support" measure.

[c]For Stage 2, this measure was incorporated into the "provide summary care document for each transition of care or referral care" measure.

[d]Reporting clinical quality measures was a meaningful use measure in Stage 1. In Stage 2, this activity is still required in order to demonstrate meaningful use, but it is not a separate meaningful use measure.

[e]Beginning in 2014, the Stage 2 criteria apply for Stage 1 with the exception that there is no requirement that patients view, download, or transmit their health information.

[f]For Stage 2, this measure was incorporated into the "provide patients with their health information electronically" measure.

[g]ONC did not indicate that this measure is related to health information exchange.
[h]This requirement was eliminated from the Stage 1 requirements beginning in 2013.
[i]For Stage 2, this measure was incorporated into the "generate and transmit permissible prescriptions electronically" measure.
[j]CMS officials did not indicate that this measure is related to the actual transfer of health information between entities. However, they noted that this measure helps enable exchange by allowing information to be structured in such a way that when it is transferred it is usable by the recipient.
[k]This requirement was eliminated from the Stage 1 requirements beginning in 2014.

APPENDIX IV: MEANINGFUL USE MEASURE REPORTING FOR THE MEDICARE EHR PROGRAM, 2011 AND 2012

In general, to receive incentive payments from the Medicare Electronic Health Record (EHR) program for 2011 or 2012, hospitals had to report on a total of 19, and professionals had to report on a total of 20, Stage 1 meaningful use measures. Among those measures reported, 14 were mandatory for hospitals and 15 were mandatory for professionals. The remaining measures were selected by providers from a list of optional measures. For certain meaningful use measures, providers must meet or exceed reporting thresholds—that is, a specified percentage of patients or actions required to satisfy the measure—established by the Centers for Medicare & Medicaid Services (CMS) and the Office of the National Coordinator for Health Information Technology (ONC) for the EHR programs. Table 6 displays the average percentage reported by providers for those measures that require providers to meet or exceed certain established thresholds. Table 7 displays the percentage of providers that reported certain measures for 2011 and 2012 but excludes from the calculation providers that reported to CMS that a measure was not relevant to them; this is referred to as claiming an exemption. Specifically, table 7 displays the percentage of providers that reported Stage 1 mandatory meaningful use measures that allow for exemptions and Stage 1 optional meaningful use measures. For 2011 and 2012, hospitals were allowed to claim exemptions from reporting 7 meaningful use measures, and professionals were allowed to claim exemptions from reporting 14 meaningful use measures.

Table 6. Average Percentage Reported by Medicare Providers for Meaningful Use Measures with Reporting Thresholds in the Electronic Health Record (EHR) Programs, by Measure, 2011 and 2012

	Mandatory (●) or optional (○) measure		Reporting threshold			Average percentage reported, by hospitals or professionals			
						Hospitals		Professionals	
Meaningful use measure	**Stage 1**	**Stage 2**	**Stage 1**	**Stage 2**	**Exchange-related**	**2011**	**2012**	**2011**	**2012**
Use computerized provider order entry (medication orders)	●	●[a]	30	60		84.3	84.4	84.0	83.2
Maintain an up-to-date problem list of current and active diagnoses	●	[b]	80	[c]		94.7	95.2	96.4	96.9
Generate and transmit permissible prescriptions electronically	● (P)	●(P) ○ (H)	40 (P)	50 (P) 10 (H)	Yes	N/A	N/A	79.1	83.1
Maintain active medication list	●	[b]	80	[c]		97.2	98.0	97.1	97.3
Maintain active medication allergy list	●	[b]	80	[c]		97.4	98.0	96.3	96.8
Record demographics	●	●	50	80		96.1	96.7	90.5	92.8
Record and chart changes in vital signs	●	●	50	80		93.1	92.5	90.2	91.8
Record smoking status for patients 13 years old or older	●	●	50	80		93.3	93.3	89.6	92.4
Provide patients with their health information electronically	●	●	50	[c]	Yes	96.4	96.2	96.3	97.3
For hospitals, provide patients with an electronic copy of discharge instructions at the time of discharge, upon request; for professionals, provide patients with clinical summaries for each office visit	●	● (P) [d](H)	50	50 (P)	Yes	95.8	94.8	78.4	81.6
Incorporate clinical lab test results into EHR as structured data	○	●	40	55	Yes[e]	95.4	95.5	91.5	92.9

	Mandatory (●) or optional (○) measure		Reporting threshold			Average percentage reported, by hospitals or professionals			
						Hospitals		Professionals	
Meaningful use measure	**Stage 1**	**Stage 2**	**Stage 1**	**Stage 2**	**Exchange-related**	**2011**	**2012**	**2011**	**2012**
Send patient reminders per patient preference for preventive or follow-up care	○ (P)	● (P)	20	[c]		N/A	N/A	61.4	64.1
Identify patient-specific education resources and provide those resources to the patient if appropriate	○	●	10	10		70.7	73.3	48.9	53.5
Perform medication reconciliation for patients received from another setting of care or provider of care	○	●	50	50	Yes[f]	84.1	85.4	89.5	90.1
Provide summary of care document for each transition or referral	○	●	50	50[g]	Yes	80.6	83.1	88.9	91.4
Record advance directives for patients 65 years or older	○ (H)	□(H)	50	50		95.5	95.8	N/A	N/A
Provide patients with timely electronic access to their health information	○[h](P)	[d]	10		Yes	N/A	N/A	72.6	75.1

Source: GAO analysis of CMS data and guidance and of information obtained from CMS and Office of the National Coordinator for Health Information Technology (ONC) officials.

Notes: Mandatory meaningful use measures are designated as (●) and optional meaningful use measures (the set of measures from which CMS allows providers the flexibility to select a subset of measures to report) as (○). Measures that apply to hospitals only are indicated by (H), and measures that apply to professionals only are indicated by (P). The "exchange-related" column identifies meaningful use measures that are related to electronic health information exchange according to CMS, ONC, or both agencies. Not applicable (N/A) indicates that the measure did not apply to that provider type.

[a]In addition to medication orders, the Stage 2 measure requires the use of computerized provider order entry for 30 percent of laboratory orders and 30 percent of radiology orders.

[b]For Stage 2, this measure was incorporated into the "provide summary of care document for each transition of care or referral" measure.

[c]The measure has changed substantially for Stage 2 such that comparison to the Stage 1 threshold is not appropriate.

[d]For Stage 2, this measure was incorporated into the "provide patients with their health information electronically" measure.

[e]CMS officials did not indicate that this measure is related to the actual transfer of health information between entities. However, they noted that this measure helps enable exchange by allowing information to be structured in such a way that when it is transferred it is usable by the recipient.

[f]ONC did not indicate that this measure is related to health information exchange.

[g]This threshold does not apply to the components of the Stage 2 measure which require that 10 percent of transitions of care and referrals be electronically transmitted and that at least one successful test of electronic exchange be conducted.

[h]This measure was eliminated from Stage 1 beginning in 2014.

Table 7. Percentage of Medicare Providers That Reported Mandatory Stage 1 Meaningful Use Measures That Allow for Exemptions or Optional Stage 1 Measures in the Electronic Health Record (EHR) Programs, by Measure, 2011 and 2012

				Percentage of providers that reported measure			
	Mandatory (●) or optional (○) measure		Exchange-related	**Hospitals**		**Professionals**	
Meaningful use measure	Stage 1	Stage 2		2011	2012	2011	2012
Mandatory Stage 1 meaningful use measures that allow for exemptions							
Use computerized provider order entry (medication orders)	●	●[a]		[b]	[b]	81.5	81.6
Generate and transmit permissible prescriptions electronically	● (P)	●(P) ○ (H)	Yes	N/A	N/A	77.5	79.4
Record and chart changes in vital signs	●	●		[b]	[b]	97.1	96.4
Record smoking status for patients 13 years old or older	●	●		99.5	99.7	99.5	99.8

				Percentage of providers that reported measure			
	Mandatory (●) or optional (○) measure		Exchange-related	**Hospitals**		**Professionals**	
Meaningful use measure	Stage 1	Stage 2		2011	2012	2011	2012
Provide patients with their health information electronically	●	●	Yes	30.4	34.5	31.2	29.4
For hospitals, provide patients with an electronic copy of discharge instructions at the time of discharge, upon request; for professionals, provide patients with clinical summaries for each office visit	●	● (P) [c](H)	Yes[d]	39.3	37.0	98.0	98.0
Optional Stage 1 meaningful use measures							
Implement drug formulary checks	○	[e]		87.4	83.0	70.4	70.3
Incorporate clinical lab test results into EHR as structured data	○	●	Yes[f]	81.2	86.1	58.4	59.7
Generate patient lists by specific conditions	○	●		100.0	100.0	75.4	70.7
Send patient reminders per patient preference for preventive or follow-up care	○ (P)	● (P)		N/A	N/A	21.3	17.2
Identify patient-specific education resources and provide those resources to the patient if appropriate	○	●		39.5	39.8	50.0	53.5
Perform medication reconciliation for patients received from another setting of care or provider of care	○	●	Yes[g]	25.6	27.3	40.7	44.2
Provide summary of care document for each transition or referral	○	●	Yes	7.6	8.0	12.8	13.2

Table 7. (Continued)

				Percentage of providers that reported measure			
	Mandatory (●) or optional (○) measure		Exchange-related	**Hospitals**		**Professionals**	
Meaningful use measure	Stage 1	Stage 2		2011	2012	2011	2012
Submit electronic data to immunization registries or immunization information systems	○	●	Yes	60.4	61.7	52.2	48.2
Submit electronic syndromic surveillance data to public health agencies	○	●(H) ○ (P)	Yes	14.0	19.8	16.1	14.5
Submit electronic data on reportable lab results to public health agencies	○ (H)	● (H)	Yes	16.3	14.8	N/A	N/A
Record advance directives for patients 65 years or older	○ (H)	○ (H)		87.0	90.6	N/A	N/A
Provide patients with timely electronic access to their health information	○[h](P)	[c]	Yes	N/A	N/A	33.4	32.6

Source: GAO analysis of CMS data and guidance and of information obtained from CMS and Office of the National Coordinator for Health Information Technology (ONC) officials.

Notes: This table provides information on the percentage of providers that reported the measure and did not claim an exemption from reporting the measure. The table does not list mandatory meaningful use measures that did not permit providers to claim exemptions from reporting since all providers were required to report those measures. Mandatory meaningful use measures are designated as (●), and optional meaningful use measures (the set of measures from which CMS allows providers the flexibility to select a subset of measures to report) as (0). Measures that apply to hospitals only are indicated by (H), and measures that apply to professionals only are indicated by (P). The "exchange-related" column identifies meaningful use measures that are related to electronic health information exchange according to CMS, ONC, or both agencies. Not applicable (N/A) indicates that the measure did not apply to that provider type.

[a]In addition to medication orders, the Stage 2 measure requires the use of computerized provider for laboratory orders and radiology orders.

[b]Hospitals were not permitted to claim an exemption from reporting the measure.

[c]For Stage 2, this measure was incorporated into the "provide patients with their health information electronically" measure.

[d]ONC did not indicate that this measure for professionals is related to health information exchange.

[e]For Stage 2, this measure was incorporated into the "generate and transmit permissible prescriptions electronically" measure.

[f]CMS officials did not indicate that this measure is related to the actual transfer of health information between entities. However, they noted that this measure helps enable exchange by allowing information to be structured in a way so that when it is transferred it is usable by the recipient.

[g]ONC did not indicate that this measure is related to health information exchange.

[h]This measure was eliminated from Stage 1 beginning in 2014.

Appendix V: Strategic Goals and Associated Performance Measures Relevant to the HER Programs

We reviewed Department of Health and Human Services (HHS), Centers for Medicare & Medicaid Services (CMS), and Office of the National Coordinator for Health Information Technology (ONC) strategic goals and categorized them into one of two major categories particularly relevant to the Electronic Health Record (EHR) programs—(1) adoption and meaningful use of EHRs; and (2) improving quality, efficiency, and patient safety.[1] The first category of goals is focused on program processes, and the second is focused on program outcomes. For the first category— adoption and meaningful use of EHRs—HHS, CMS, and ONC have established 26 performance measures. See table 8 for the department- and agency-level strategic goals and performance measures that fall into this category.

Note that ONC has three other goals that are relevant to the EHR programs but did not fall into the two categories we focused on and are thus not included in the table. Similarly to the measures identified in table 8, the performance measures associated with those additional goals enable the agency to track processes but not outcomes.[2]

Table 8. Department- and Agency-Level Strategic Goals and Associated Performance Measures Related to "Adoption and Meaningful Use of Electronic Health Records"

Department and/or agency	Strategic goal	Associated measures
HHS	Promote the adoption and meaningful use of health information technology (HIT)	Number of eligible providers who receive an incentive payment from the CMSMedicare and Medicaid Electronic Health Record (EHR) Incentive Programs for the successful adoption or meaningful use of certified EHR technology Percentage of office-based primary care physicians who have adopted EHRs

Department and/or agency	Strategic goal	Associated measures
Office of the National Coordinator for Health Information Technology (ONC)	Achieve adoption and information exchange through meaningful use of HIT	Percentage of office-based physicians who have adopted EHRs Percentage of office-based primary care physicians who have adopted EHRs Percentage of nonfederal acute care hospitals that have adopted EHRs Percentage of eligible hospitals receiving meaningful use incentive payments Percentage of eligible professionals receiving meaningful use incentive payments Number of eligible providers who receive an incentive payment from the CMSMedicare and Medicaid EHR Incentive Programs for the successful adoption or meaningful use of certified EHR technology EHR adoption rate among providers registered and working with ONC Regional Extension Centers for at least 10 months Number of providers registered with ONC Regional Extension Centers that achieve meaningful use Percentage of community pharmacies that are capable of exchanging health information electronically Percentage of providers prescribing through an EHR Percentage of office-based physicians who are electronically sharing any patient health information with other providers Percentage of office-based physicians who are electronically sharing patient information with any providers outside their organization Percentage of office-based physicians who are electronically sharing information using a Summary Care Record Percentage of nonfederal acute care hospitals that are electronically exchanging patient health information with any providers outside their organization Percentage of nonfederal acute care hospitals that are electronically sharing clinical/summary care records with any providers outside their organization

Table 8. (Continued)

Department and/or agency	Strategic goal	Associated measures
		Percentage of nonfederal acute care hospitals that are electronically sharing any patient health information with ambulatory providers outside their organization Percentage of eligible hospitals that have adopted EHRs Percentage of Federally Qualified Health Centers that are affiliated with providers that receive Medicare and Medicaid EHR incentive programs payments
CMS	Expanding the use of EHRs through the concept of meaningful use	Number of eligible professionals receiving EHR incentive payments for the successful demonstration of meaningful use for Medicare Number of eligible professionals receiving EHR incentive payments for the successful demonstration of meaningful use under Medicaid Number of eligible hospitals and critical access hospitals receiving EHR incentive payments for the successful demonstration of meaningful use underMedicare Number of eligible hospitals and critical access hospitals receiving EHR incentive payments for the successful demonstration of meaningful use underMedicaid Number of eligible professionals receiving EHR incentive payments for adopt/implement/upgrade under the Medicaid incentive program Number of eligible hospitals receiving EHR incentive payments for adopt/implement/upgrade under the Medicaid incentive program

Source: GAO analysis of agency HHS, CMS, and ONC information.

Note: HHS, CMS, and ONC have not established performance measures for the EHR programs for the second category—improving quality, efficiency, and patient safety, focused on program outcomes. See table 9 for the department- and agency-level strategic goals that fall into this category.

Table 9. Department- and Agency-Level Strategic Goals Related to "Improving Quality, Efficiency, and Patient Safety"

Department and/or agency	Strategic goals
HHS	Improve health care quality and patient safety Reduce the growth of health care costs while promoting high-value, effective care
Office of the National Coordinator for Health Information Technology (ONC)	Improve care, improve population health, and reduce health care costs through the useof health information technology
CMS	Improve health care quality, efficiency, and patient safety

Source: GAO analysis of agency HHS, CMS, and ONC information.

APPENDIX VI: PROGRAM EVALUATIONS ASSESSING THE EHR PROGRAMS' EFFECTS ON OUTCOMES

Centers for Medicare & Medicaid Services (CMS) and Office of the National Coordinator for Health Information Technology (ONC) officials told us they are conducting some evaluations to assess the effect of the Electronic Health Record (EHR) programs on outcomes. See table 10 for a summary of these evaluations according to agency officials.

Table 10. Summary of Program Evaluations Assessing the Electronic Health Record (EHR) Programs on Outcomes

Evaluation description	Data source	Status
Analysis of the association between the use of e-prescribing and adverse drug events	Medicare Part D claims	Expected peer review in early 2014
Analysis of the association between health information technology and hospital quality	Health information technology infrastructure data from the American Hospital Association and CMS's National Level Repository[a]; Hospital quality data from Hospital Compare[b]	Compiling analytic data files

Table 10. (Continued)

Evaluation description	Data source	Status
Analysis of the extent to which laboratories have the capability to send results back to physicians and the extent to which they are doing so	Survey of laboratories conducted by NORC	Survey completed; compiling analytic data files. Preliminary data expected early 2014
Analysis of whether physicians report that using EHRs provides improved patient care overall or specific clinical benefits and whether benefits depend on participating in the EHR programs or length of EHR experience	Physician Workflow Survey	Accepted for publication in Health Services Research
Analysis of EHR adopters versus nonadopters and their perceptions of the benefits of using EHRs	Physician Workflow Survey	Under peer review
A global evaluation of the State Health Information Exchange Cooperative Agreement Program, the Regional Extension Center Program, the Beacon Communities Program, and the Information Technology Professionals in Health Care to assess the overall impact of the four programs on adoption and meaningful use of EHRs and on resulting changes in health quality and cost[c]	Medicare claims	Developing analysis plan and obtaining data; final report expected in March 2015
Analysis of changes in quality, efficiency, and population health measures in Beacon Communities, comparing provider participants and nonparticipants[c]	Medicare claims	Developing analysis plan and obtaining data; final report expected in early 2015
Literature review on the impact of EHRs on outcomes	Published literature	Published in Annals of InternalMedicine on January 7, 2014[d]

Source: GAO analysis of CMS and Office of the National Coordinator for Health Information Technology (ONC) information.

[a]CMS collects data about the Medicare and Medicaid EHR programs in the National Level Repository.

[b]Hospital Compare is a CMS website that publicly reports clinical quality measures by hospital.

[c]The State Health Information Exchange Cooperative Agreement Program promotes health information exchange that will advance mechanisms for information sharing across the health care system. The Regional Extension Center program provides assistance to providers such as professionals in solo practices or rural areas to help them participate in the EHR programs. The Beacon Communities Program funds 17 selected communities throughout the United States to build and strengthen health information technology (HIT) infrastructure and exchange capabilities within communities, to translate investments in HIT to measureable improvements in outcomes, and to develop innovative approaches to performance measurement, technology, and care delivery. Information Technology Professionals in Health Care funds the training and development of a workforce that will meet short-term programmatic needs related to the Health Information Technology for Economic and Clinical Health (HITECH) Act.

[d]See Spencer S. Jones, Robert S. Rudin, Tanja Perry, and Paul G. Shekelle, "Health Information Technology: An Updated Systematic Review with a Focus on Meaningful Use," *Annals of Internal Medicine*, vol. 160, no. 1 (2014).

End Notes

[1] See Pub. L. No. 111-5, §§ 4101-4201, 123 Stat. 115, 467-494. Medicare is a federal program financing health care for individuals age 65 and older, certain disabled individuals, and individuals with end-stage renal disease. In 2012, Medicare covered over 49 million beneficiaries. Medicaid is a federal-state program financing health care for certain low-income individuals. In fiscal year 2011, Medicaid covered about 70 million beneficiaries.

[2] See C.J. Hsiao, E. Hing, T.C. Socey, and B. Cai, "Electronic Medical Record/Electronic Health Record Systems of Office-Based Physicians: United States, 2009 and Preliminary 2010 State Estimates," *National Center for Health Statistics Health E-stat* (2010); and A.K. Jha, C.M. DesRoches, P.D. Kralovec, and M.S. Joshi, "A Progress Report On Electronic Health Records In U.S. Hospitals," *Health Affairs*, no.10 (2010):1951-1957.

[3] The HITECH Act was enacted as title XIII of division A and title IV of division B of the American Recovery and Reinvestment Act of 2009. Pub. L. No 111-5, div. A, tit. XIII, 123 Stat. 115, 226-279 and div. B, tit. IV, 123 Stat. 115, 467-496 (2009). The HITECH Act created incentive programs for Medicare fee-for-service, Medicare Advantage, and Medicaid. Under the Medicare Advantage EHR program, Medicare Advantage Organizations—private companies that provide Medicare health insurance coverage to beneficiaries for hospital, physician, and other services—receive incentive payments for certain affiliated professionals and hospitals that meet program requirements. Pub. L. No. 111-5, §§ 4101(c), 4102(c), 123 Stat. 473-476, 484-486. In this report we focus primarily on the Medicare fee-for-service EHR program, which we refer to as the Medicare EHR program, and the Medicaid EHR program. Other activities funded by the HITECH Act

include, for example, grants to Regional Extension Centers to assist certain providers, such as physicians in small primary care practices, with adopting, implementing, and meaningfully using EHRs; and assistance to higher education institutions to establish or expand medical health informatics education programs.

[4] Congressional Budget Office, "Health Information Technology for Economic and Clinical Health Act" (Washington, D.C.: Jan. 21, 2009). This estimate includes spending estimates for bonuses and payment reductions from the penalties.

[5] Providers permitted to participate vary by program. Permissible hospitals under the Medicare EHR program are acute care hospitals described in Section 1886(d) of the Social Security Act, which are paid under the inpatient prospective payment system in the 50 states and the District of Columbia; and critical access hospitals. Permissible hospitals under the Medicaid EHR program are acute care hospitals, critical access hospitals, cancer hospitals, and children's hospitals. Permissible professionals under the Medicare EHR program are doctors of medicine or osteopathy, doctors of dental surgery or dental medicine, doctors of podiatry, doctors of optometry, and chiropractors. Permissible professionals under the Medicaid EHR program are doctors of medicine or osteopathy, doctors of dental surgery or dental medicine, nurse practitioners, certified nurse-midwives, and physician assistants who furnish services in a federally qualified health center or rural health clinic that is led by a physician assistant.

[6] See Pub. L. No. 111-5, § 4101(a)-(b), 123 Stat. 467-473.

[7] See Pub. L. No 111-5, § 4101 (a) 123 Stat. 467-472, 477-485.

[8] See Medicare and Medicaid Programs: Electronic Health Record Incentive Program, 75 Fed. Reg. 44314 (July 28, 2010), codified at 42 C.F.R. pts. 412, 413, 422 and 495; Health Information Technology: Initial Set of Standards, Implementation Specifications, and Certification Criteria for Electronic Health Records Technology, 75 Fed. Reg. 44590 (July 28, 2010), codified at 45 C.F.R. pt. 170; Medicare and Medicaid Programs; Electronic Health Record Incentive Program—Stage 2, 77 Fed. Reg. 53968 (Sept. 4, 2012), codified at 42 C.F.R. pts. 412, 413, and 495; and Health Information Technology: Standards, Implementation Specifications, and Certification Criteria for Electronic Health Records Technology, 2014 Edition, 77 Fed. Reg. 54163 (Sept. 4, 2012), codified at 45 C.F.R. pt. 170.

[9] CMS provides states with 100 percent of the cost of incentive payments made to Medicaid providers and 90 percent of the costs related to reasonable administrative expenses and planning activities related to the Medicaid EHR program. 42 U.S.C. § 1396b(a)(3)(F)(i) and (ii).

[10] To receive incentive payments from the EHR programs, providers must use certified EHR technology.

[11] Pub.L. No. 111-5, § 13001, 123 Stat. 230-234.

[12] Pub.L. No. 111-5, § 13424(e), 123 Stat. 278-279.

[13] See GAO, *Electronic Health Records: First Year of CMS's Incentive Programs Shows Opportunities to Improve Processes to Verify Providers Met Requirements*, GAO-12-481 (Washington, D.C.: Apr. 30, 2012).

[14] See GAO, *Electronic Health Records: Number and Characteristics of Providers Awarded Medicare Incentive Payments for 2011*, GAO-12-778R (Washington, D.C.: July 26, 2012).

[15] GAO, *Electronic Health Records: Number and Characteristics of Providers Awarded Medicaid Incentive Payments for 2011*, GAO-13-146R (Washington, D.C.: Dec. 13, 2012).

[16] GAO, *Electronic Health Records: Number and Characteristics of Providers Awarded Medicare Incentive Payments for 2011–2012*, GAO-14-21R (Washington, D.C.: Oct. 24, 2013).

[17] In this report, we use the term "participation" to mean providers awarded incentive payments for meeting the requirements of either the Medicare or the Medicaid (or, in the case of some hospitals, both) EHR program.

At the time of our analysis, according to CMS, 14 states and the District of Columbia had not completed their determinations of which providers would receive incentive payments for the 2012 program year. As a result, our analyses of the Medicaid EHR program do not reflect payments incorporated into CMS's National Level Repository after October 23, 2013.

[18] For the Medicaid EHR program, we limited this analysis to providers that were awarded incentive payments from 36 states that, according to CMS, had completed their determinations of which providers would receive incentive payments for the 2011 and 2012 Medicaid EHR program years as of October 23, 2013.

[19] An exclusion for a nonapplicable measure is permitted if the provider meets certain requirements specified in the regulation. 42 C.F.R. § 495.6. In this report, we use the term "exemption" to refer to the exclusion of a nonapplicable measure. The agency allows providers to claim exemptions from reporting certain meaningful use measures to help ensure that providers with all types of patient populations and clinical practices could potentially demonstrate meaningful use. See 75 Fed. Reg. 44328-44329 (July 28, 2010). For 2011 and 2012, hospitals were permitted to claim exemptions from reporting 7 meaningful use measures, and professionals from reporting 14 meaningful use measures.

[20] See Medicare Program; Hospital Inpatient Prospective Payment Systems for Acute Care Hospitals and the Long Term Care; Hospital Prospective Payment System and Fiscal Year 2014 Rates; Quality Reporting Requirements for Specific Providers; Hospital Conditions of Participation; Payment Policies Related to Patient Status, 78 Fed. Reg. 50496 (August 19, 2013), codified at 42 C.F.R. pts. 412, 413, 414, 419, 424, 482, 485 and 489; and Medicare Program; Revisions to Payment Policies Under the Physician Fee Schedule, Clinical Laboratory Fee Schedule & Other Revisions to Part B for CY 2014, 78 Fed. Reg. 74230 (December 10, 2013), codified at 42 C.F.R. pts. 405, 410, 411, 414, 423 and 425.

[21] See GAO, *Government Operations: Internal Control Management and Evaluation Tool (Supersedes* GAO-01-131G*),* GAO-01-1008G (Washington, D.C.: Aug. 1, 2001).

[22] Measures that capture a small number of patients may be unreliable measures of quality because relatively small changes in the number of patients who experienced the care processes or outcomes targeted by the measure can generate large shifts in the calculated percentage for the measure.

[23] See Pub. L. No. 111-352, 124 Stat. 3866 (Jan. 4, 2011). GPRAMA amends the Government Performance and Results Act of 1993, Pub. L. No. 103-62, 107 Stat. 285 (1993); GAO, *Executive Guide: Effectively Implementing the Government Performance and Results Act,* GAO/GGD-96-118 (Washington, D.C.: June 1, 1996); and GAO, *Designing Evaluations: 2012 Revision,* GAO-12-208G (Washington, D.C.: January 31, 2012).

[24] References in this report to a year conform to the concept of program year, which for hospitals is based on the fiscal year and for professionals is based on the calendar year. For example, for hospitals, the 2011 program year was from October 1, 2010, to September 30, 2011, whereas for professionals, the 2011 program year was from January 1, 2011, to December 31, 2011.

[25] We previously reported that the median payments to hospitals in the Medicare EHR program and Medicaid EHR program for 2011 were $1.6 million and $613,512, respectively. See GAO-14-21R and GAO-13-146R.

[26] CMS will increase the incentive payments that would otherwise apply by 10 percent each year for Medicare professionals who predominantly furnish services in geographic areas designated as health professional shortage areas, such as areas that have a shortage of primary medical care.

[27] Most providers must meet program requirements prior to the start of the 2015 program year in order to avoid penalties from the Medicare EHR program. For example, professionals first participating in 2014 must meet the requirements in the first 9 months of calendar year 2014 to avoid penalties in 2015. In general, providers must continue to demonstrate meaningful use each year to avoid penalties in later years.

[28] For example, if the increase to the Medicare Inpatient Prospective Payment System payment rate in 2015 was 2 percent, then an acute care hospital that did not meet Medicare EHR program requirements would only receive a 1.5 percent increase that year.

[29] For 2018 and each subsequent year, if CMS finds that less than 75 percent of professionals meet the Medicare EHR Program's requirements, CMS may increase the penalty percentage in the Medicare EHR Program beginning in 2018 by up to 1 percent per year, with a maximum cumulative penalty of up to 5 percent per year. See 42 U.S.C. §§ 1395w-4(a)(7)(A)(iii).

[30] See 42 U.S.C. §§ 1395w-4(a)(7)(B).

[31] For the Medicaid EHR program, hospitals must generally have a Medicaid patient volume of at least 10 percent and professionals must generally have a Medicaid patient volume of at least 30 percent.

[32] See Pub.L. No. 111-5, § 4201, 123 Stat. 493.

[33] In this report, when we use the term EHR, we are generally referring to certified EHR technology.

[34] ONC is planning to issue an interim set of standards and certification criteria (2015- edition) intended to be responsive to stakeholder feedback and to address issues found in the 2014-edition EHRs. These standards would be optional—providers participating in the EHR programs would not be required to use EHRs certified using the interim criteria.

[35] HHS regulations specify the stage that is applicable to a provider in each year. The start of Stage 2, which was originally expected to begin in 2013, was delayed by HHS for 1 year due to concerns expressed by providers and in response to recommendations from the HIT Policy Committee, which advises ONC on HIT policy. As a result of this change, the start of Stage 3 would have been 2016; however, on December 6, 2013, CMS announced that the start of Stage 3 would be pushed back to 2017.

[36] In this example, by demonstrating meaningful use for 2013 and 2014, the professional would also avoid penalties for 2015 and 2016, respectively.

[37] According to ONC, the Stage 2 meaningful use measures require the use of more specific interoperability standards, which are incorporated into 2014-edition EHRs.

[38] For example, the CQM that measures use of high-risk medications in the elderly comprises the following data elements—the number of patients with a medication order for at least one high-risk medication and at least two high-risk medications during the measurement period and the number of patients treated by the professional. Two scores are then calculated by (1) dividing the number of patients with at least one medication by the number of patients treated, and (2) dividing the number of patients with at least two medications by the number of patients treated.

[39] In 2012, we reported on activities conducted by the National Quality Forum under contract with HHS, including efforts to modify CQMs so they could be collected using EHRs. See GAO, *Health Care Quality Measurement: HHS Should Address Contractor Performance and Plan for Needed Measures,* GAO-12-136 (Washington, D.C.: Jan. 13, 2012). The National Quality Forum is the entity in the United States with the lead responsibility for endorsing CQMs.

[40] Professionals had to report 3 core or alternative core measures and had to report an additional 3 measures from the list of measures.

[41] Hospitals and professionals must report CQMs that cover at least three of the following six domains, which are based on the six National Quality Strategy priorities: patient and family engagement; patient safety; care coordination; population and public health; efficient use of healthcare resources; and clinical processes or effectiveness.

[42] For the 2012 and 2013 program years, providers were permitted but not required to submit CQM data to CMS electronically for the Medicare EHR program through electronic reporting pilot programs—one for hospitals and one for professionals. For 2012, no hospitals and less than 2 percent of professionals who received incentive payments submitted CQM data to CMS electronically for the Medicare EHR program through a pilot in order to demonstrate meaningful use. CMS is working with the states to develop capabilities to receive electronically submitted CQM results from providers for the Medicaid EHR program.

[43] See Pub. L. No. 111-148, §§ 3007, 3022, 124 Stat. 119, 373-376, 395-399 (2010). In its quality reporting programs, CMS gives consideration to CQMs that have been endorsed by the National Quality Forum.

[44] Hospitals choosing this option would have to report data for the remaining IQR measures using the traditional manual data collection techniques that are based on chart abstraction.

[45] Professionals choosing this option must report CQMs from the list of 64 CQMs identified for the EHR programs. To meet the criteria for satisfactory reporting to PQRS, professionals must report at least 1 CQM with at least one patient in the denominator of the measure. Additionally, professionals must report CQM data collected over the 12-month period required by PQRS instead of the 3-month period required by the EHR programs in 2014.
Professionals submitting CQM data generated from 2014-edition EHRs to "qualified" clinical data registries in 2014—established under a new program enacted under the American Taxpayer Relief Act of 2012—will also satisfy the CQM reporting requirements for both PQRS and the Medicare EHR program. In 2013, we reported on HHS's plans for this new program and recommended several actions that HHS could take to help ensure that qualified clinical data registries promote improved quality and efficiency of physician care for Medicare beneficiaries. See GAO, *Clinical Data Registries: HHS Could Improve Medicare Quality and Efficiency through Key Requirements and Oversight*, GAO-14-75 (Washington, D.C.: Dec. 16, 2013).

[46] By 2017, the Physician Value Based Payment Modifier will apply regardless of the professional's practice size.

[47] GAO, *Performance Measurement and Evaluation: Definitions and Relationships*, GAO-11-646SP (Washington, D.C.: May 2, 2011).

[48] GAO, *Executive Guide: Effectively Implementing the Government Performance and Results Act*, GAO/GGD-96-118 (Washington, D.C.: June 1, 1996).

[49] GAO, *Designing Evaluations: 2012 Revision,* GAO-12-208G (Washington, D.C.: Jan. 31, 2012).

[50] Only a subset of providers that participated in the Medicaid EHR programs for 2011 and 2012 demonstrated meaningful use. For the Medicaid EHR program, providers are not required to demonstrate meaningful use for their first year of participation; they need only report that they adopted, implemented, or upgraded to EHRs. Of the providers that participated in the Medicaid EHR program in 2011, 27 percent of hospitals and less than 1 percent of professionals demonstrated meaningful use. Of the providers that participated in the Medicaid EHR program in 2012, 73 percent of hospitals and 29 percent of professionals demonstrated meaningful use.

[51] An additional 31 hospitals participated in the Medicare Advantage EHR program for 2011, and an additional 32 hospitals did so for 2012.

[52] An additional 11,137 professionals participated in the Medicare Advantage EHR program for 2011, and an additional 11,340 professionals did so for 2012.

[53] CMS paid an additional $232 million in incentive payments to providers for participating in the Medicare Advantage EHR program for 2011 and an additional $180 million to providers for participating in the Medicare Advantage EHR program for 2012, for a total of $412 million for both years—$96 million of which was paid for hospitals' participation and the remaining $316 million for professionals' participation.

[54] Prior to the implementation of the EHR programs, CMS estimated (in its final rule for Stage 1 of meaningful use) the total payments that would be awarded to providers during fiscal year 2011 and fiscal year 2012, with a low estimate of $3.4 billion and a high estimate of $8.6 billion. These estimates were based on fiscal year payments and cannot be directly compared with the payments reported above, which are based on program years and not when the payments were made. Thus, we also determined total payments awarded to providers during fiscal year 2011 and fiscal year 2012: a total of $7.6 billion was awarded to providers during fiscal years 2011 and 2012, which is lower than CMS's high estimate

[55] At the time of our analysis, according to CMS, 14 states and the District of Columbia had not completed their determinations of which providers would receive incentive payments for the 2011 and 2012 Medicaid EHR program years. As a result, to calculate the percentage of professionals and the percentage of hospitals that participated in the Medicaid EHR program in 2011 but did not continue in 2012, we excluded those states that had not completed their determinations.

[56] To receive incentive payments, providers that demonstrated meaningful use for the first time in 2011 and 2012 must meet Stage 2 requirements for demonstrating meaningful use starting in 2014. Providers that demonstrated meaningful use for the first time in 2013 or 2014 must meet Stage 2 requirements starting in 2015 and 2016, respectively.

[57] Specifically, an analysis of the American Hospital Association's 2012 survey of hospitals indicates that 5.1 percent of acute care hospitals could meet all 16 of the mandatory meaningful use measures for Stage 2. See C.M. DesRoches, D. Charles, M.F. Furukawa, M.S. Joshi, P. Kralovec, F. Mostashari, C. Worzala, and A.K. Jha, "Adoption of Electronic Health Records Grows Rapidly, but Fewer Than Half of US Hospitals Had at Least a Basic System in 2012," *Health Affairs*, no. 32 (2013): 1478-1485.

[58] To avoid penalties in 2015, most eligible providers who first demonstrated meaningful use in 2011 or 2012 were required to do so again for a full year in 2013. Otherwise, by first demonstrating meaningful use in 2013 or in 2014 (that is, by July 1, 2014, for hospitals or October 1, 2014, for professionals), eligible providers could avoid penalties in 2015. In general, providers must continue to demonstrate meaningful use each year to avoid penalties in subsequent years.

[59] ONC funding to Regional Extension Centers—approximately $721 million in grants—will not be available after 2015. ONC indicated that Regional Extension Centers will continue to provide services to providers but anticipates that the scope and scale of these services will be dramatically reduced.

[60] See GAO-14-21R. Although participation among rural hospitals and solo practitioners grew rapidly, for 2011 and 2012, hospitals in urban areas and professionals in larger practices were more likely to have participated in the Medicare EHR program.

[61] In general, hospital-based professionals are not eligible to receive incentive payments or incur penalties from the Medicare and Medicaid EHR programs. A hospital-based professional is a professional who performs 90 percent or more of his or her services in the prior year in hospital inpatient or emergency room settings.

[62] For meaningful use measures with reporting thresholds, those thresholds ranged from 10 to 80 percent. See app. III for a list of the meaningful use measures and, if applicable, the thresholds established for them for Stage 1.

[63] Similarly to our finding for hospitals, of the 16 professional meaningful use measures that had thresholds, on average, professionals reported rates at least 10 percentage points above the measures' thresholds for all measures and exceeded thresholds by considerably more for many measures. For example, professionals were required to provide patients with timely electronic access to their health information for at least 10 percent of patients. For both 2011 and 2012, professionals reported doing so for more than 70 percent of their patients.

[64] A CMS analysis of professionals who received incentive payments from the Medicaid EHR program for 2012 for demonstrating meaningful use—approximately 30 percent of professionals in the program—provides evidence that those Medicaid professionals consistently exceeded required thresholds. These professionals exceeded thresholds by at least 15 percentage points for all measures and by considerably more for many measures. CMS analyzed data it received from states on measures Medicaid professionals reported to demonstrate meaningful use for 2012, the first year during which some Medicaid providers were required to demonstrate meaningful use to receive a Medicaid EHR incentive payment. These data have limitations. For example, according to CMS officials, states reported data on only a subset of Medicaid professionals who demonstrated meaningful use in 2012 and we do not know how representative this sample is of all professionals who received incentive payments from the Medicaid EHR program for 2012 for demonstrating meaningful use.

[65] For Stage 2, CMS increased the reporting thresholds from the Stage 1 thresholds for five hospital measures and six professional measures. Other Stage 1 measures with thresholds do not have more stringent Stage 2 thresholds, changed substantially for Stage 2 such that a comparison to the Stage 1 thresholds is not appropriate, or are not Stage 2 measures.

[66] For certain measures, providers were not required to report mandatory and optional measures that were not relevant to them—which is referred to as claiming an exemption— and were only required to choose a subset of optional measures to report. In Stage 1, hospitals were permitted to claim exemptions from reporting three mandatory measures and four optional measures, and professionals were permitted to claim exemptions from reporting six mandatory measures and eight optional measures. (See app. III for the measures for which exemptions are permitted.)

[67] Other measures not related to the electronic exchange of information may also be problematic for providers. For example, fewer than 25 percent of Medicare professionals in 2011 and 2012 reported sending patient reminders for preventive or follow-up care. This measure is optional for professionals in Stage 1 and mandatory for professionals in Stage 2.

[68] The reportable lab results measure is not a measure for professionals in either stage.

[69] Ongoing submission is also necessary in Stage 2 to meet requirements of the following exchange-related public health measures, the last two of which are new for professionals in Stage 2: immunization data, cancer cases, and other specific cases.

[70] In the previously mentioned CMS analysis, among the mandatory meaningful use measures reported by the approximately 30 percent of professionals who received incentive payments from the Medicaid EHR program for 2012 for demonstrating meaningful use, this measure was the least frequently reported.

[71] See DesRoches et al., "Adoption of Electronic Health Records," 1482. The survey asked whether hospitals had implemented specific clinical functions that may be part of an EHR system and that are related to many of the capabilities required to demonstrate Stage 1 and Stage 2 meaningful use. The study authors considered the capability to have been implemented if the hospital's system had the capability or had implemented it in at least one hospital unit.

[72] 78 Fed. Reg. 14793 (March 7, 2013).

[73] See *Principles and Strategy for Accelerating Health Information Exchange (HIE)*. Office of the National Coordinator for Health Information Technology and the Centers for Medicare & Medicaid Services. August 7, 2013.

[74] In 2012, we recommended that HHS test CQMs to help identify potential errors and address issues of implementation. See GAO-12-136. HHS implemented our recommendation by having various CMS contractors complete feasibility testing of new measures incorporated into 2014-edition EHRs and by establishing plans to test future measures.

[75] The data elements associated with each CQM collected using certified EHRs include lists of specific values that define clinical concepts (e.g., patient with diabetes, clinical visits, and reportable diseases) and are used to define the patient populations that should be included in the computation of CQMs.

[76] Testing bodies use the certification testing tool—Cypress—to test that EHRs accurately export, calculate, and electronically submit the data. This tool includes synthetic patient data used in the testing process. Vendors also have access to the testing tool prior to submitting their EHR products for certification.

[77] To qualify for incentive payments from the Medicare EHR program for the 2014 program year, the deadline for submitting CQM data to CMS is November 30, 2014, for hospitals and February 28, 2015, for professionals.

[78] ONC officials said that the agency releases new versions of the certification testing tool for various reasons, including to address mistakes, to reflect changes to the specifications, and to improve the tool.

[79] CMS is taking steps to address this issue in some of its programs that use CQMs. For example, the Physician Value Based Payment Modifier will include only CQMs that are based on a minimum of 20 patients. In addition, the agency's Hospital Compare website, which publicly reports CQMs by hospital, indicates whether the number of patients included in a particular measure calculation was based on fewer than 25 patients and was thus too small to reliably tell how well the hospital is performing.

[80] We defined few as fewer than 7 patients for providers who submitted data collected over a 90-day reporting period and as fewer than 25 patients for providers who submitted data collected over a full-year reporting period. The reporting period is generally 90 days for the first year a provider demonstrates meaningful use and a full year thereafter.

Our analysis included all patients reported by the provider, irrespective of insurance type. The likelihood that professionals who satisfy the Medicare EHR program's CQM requirements by reporting through PQRS will report measures based on few patients could be greater, because these professionals report CQMs only on Medicare patients.

[81] For the 2012 and 2013 program years, providers were permitted but not required to submit CQM data to CMS electronically through electronic reporting pilot programs—one for hospitals and one for professionals.

[82] GAO has previously reported on CMS's efforts to ensure the reliability of hospital quality data collected for the IQR program. See GAO, *Hospital Quality Data: CMS Needs More Rigorous Methods to Ensure Reliability of Publicly Released Data,* GAO-06-54 (Washington, D.C.: Jan. 31, 2006).

[83] GAO, *Executive Guide: Effectively Implementing the Government Performance and Results Act*, GAO/GGD-96-118 (Washington, D.C.: June 1, 1996).

[84] In addition, the Centers for Disease Control and Prevention has 3 performance measures related to the meaningful use of EHRs intended to measure the readiness of public health agencies to receive electronically submitted data as part of the EHR programs. The Centers for Disease Control and Prevention provides direct assistance to state public health agencies to support electronic health information systems to receive data from providers.

[85] For instance, see Department of Health and Human Services, *Fiscal Year 2014: Office of the National Coordinator for Health Information Technology Justification of Estimates for Appropriations Committee* (Washington, D.C.), accessed April 11, 2013, http://www.healthit.gov/newsroom/onc-budget-documents-and-performance-information.

[86] In July 2013, ONC published a plan to strengthen patient safety efforts across government programs and the private sector. This plan outlines efforts to collect information on patient safety such as aggregate data on HIT-related adverse events and hazards and calls for the agency to develop performance measures for patient safety. See the Office of the National Coordinator for Health Information Technology, *Health IT Patient Safety Action & Surveillance Plan* (July 2, 2013), accessed August 14, 2013, www.healthit.gov/sites/default /files/safety_plan_master.pdf.

[87] CMS's Medicare Part D provides outpatient prescription drug benefits for Medicare beneficiaries.

End Notes for Appendix I

[1] Three of the four health insurance companies we contacted were listed in the top 25 health insurance companies as ranked by US News & World Report, based on nationwide market share.

[2] The medical loss ratio is a basic financial indicator, traditionally referring to the percentage of premiums spent on medical claims.

End Notes for Appendix II

[1] For the Medicare and Medicaid EHR programs, program years are determined and awarded on a fiscal year basis for hospitals and on a calendar year basis for professionals.

[2] The total number of providers that received Medicare EHR incentive payments for 2011 or 2012 and the total amount of incentive payments awarded for either year could change due to provider audits or appeals.

[3] Using a similar approach, we determined the number of providers that met the participation requirements of the Medicare Advantage EHR program for both years.

[4] See 75 Fed. Reg. 44314, 44548 (July 28, 2010).

[5] Using a similar approach, we determined the total amount awarded from the Medicare Advantage EHR program for both years.

We also determined the total amount awarded to providers from the Medicare, Medicaid, and Medicare Advantage EHR programs for fiscal year 2011 and fiscal year 2012 by using the date the payment was made to sum the payments awarded to providers in each fiscal year.

[6] Providers that had a Medicare EHR program incentive payment disbursed to them for 2011 and a Medicaid EHR program incentive payment disbursed to them for 2012, or vice versa, were included in our determination of providers awarded EHR incentive payments both years.

[7] For 2012, no hospitals and less than 2 percent of professionals who received incentive payments submitted CQM data to the electronic reporting pilots to demonstrate meaningful use.

[8] Specifically, in Stage 1, hospitals were permitted to claim exemptions from reporting three mandatory measures and four optional measures, and professionals were permitted to claim exemptions from reporting six mandatory measures and eight optional measures.

[9] Some CQMs are composed of more than one submeasure. In these cases, we analyzed the submeasure for which providers reported the greatest number of patients in the denominator of the measure.

[10] See J. King, V. Patel, and M. Furukawa, "Physician Adoption of Electronic Health Record Technology to Meet Meaningful Use Objectives: 2009-2012," ONC Data Brief, no. 7 (Washington, D.C.: Office of the National Coordinator for Health Information Technology, December 2012).

End Note for Appendix III

[1] Except for 2014, providers must collect data related to the meaningful use measures in any 90 consecutive days in their first year of reporting meaningful use and for a full year in subsequent years. For 2014 only, all providers, regardless of their stage of meaningful use, are required to collect data related to the meaningful use measures for only 3 months.

In the Medicare and Medicaid EHR programs, professionals include doctors of medicine and dental surgery. In the Medicaid EHR program, professionals also include nurse practitioners, certified nurse-midwives, and certain physician assistants.

CMS made some changes to the Stage 1 requirements that apply after 2012. For example, one mandatory meaningful use measure was eliminated from the requirements in Stage 1 beginning in the 2013 program year.

End Notes for Appendix V

[1] There are other goals that we determined were not relevant to the EHR programs. For example, HHS has a goal to advance scientific knowledge and innovation, which includes the objective to invest in the regulatory sciences to improve food and medical product safety. A full list of strategic goals and associated performance measures can be found in the following: HHS, *U.S. Department of Health and Human Services Fiscal Years 2010 2015 Strategic Plan* (Washington, D.C.), accessed April 19, 2013, http://www.hhs.gov/secretary/about/priorities/strategicplan2010-2015.pdf; ONC, *Federal Health Information Technology Strategic Plan, 2011-2015* (Washington, D.C.), accessed December 6, 2012, http://www.healthit.gov/sites/default/files/utility/final-federal-health-it-strategic-plan-0911.pd f; and the EHR programs' requirements (found in CMS's Stage 1 and Stage 2 final rules), as well as HHS, *Fiscal Year 2014 Annual Performance Report and Performance Plan* (Apr. 2013), accessed April 19, 2013, http://www.hhs.gov/budget/fy2014/opa_040513.pdf; HHS, *Fiscal Year 2014 Centers for Medicare & Medicaid Services Justification of Estimates for Appropriations Committee* (Baltimore, MD), accessed April 19, 2013, http://www.cms.gov/about-cms/agencyinformation/performancebudget/index.html?redirect=/performancebudget/; and HHS, *Fiscal Year 2014: Office of the National Coordinator for the Health Information Technology Justification of Estimates for Appropriations Committee* (Washington, D.C.), accessed April 11, 2013, http://www.healt hit.gov/newsroom/onc-budget-documents-and-performance-information.

[2] The three goals are to inspire confidence and trust in health information technology (HIT); to empower individuals with HIT to improve their health and the health care system; and to achieve rapid learning and technical advancement. See ONC, *Federal Health Information Technology Strategic Plan, 2011-2015.*

In: Electronic Health Records
Editor: Carole Medina
ISBN: 978-1-63482-276-3

Chapter 2

ELECTRONIC HEALTH RECORDS: HHS STRATEGY TO ADDRESS INFORMATION EXCHANGE CHALLENGES LACKS SPECIFIC PRIORITIZED ACTIONS AND MILESTONES*

United States Government Accountability Office

ABBREVIATIONS

ACO	accountable care organization
AHA	American Hospital Association
CCD	continuity of care document
CHIME	College of Healthcare Information Management Executives
CMS	Centers for Medicare & Medicaid Services
EHR	electronic health record
GPRA	Government Performance and Results Act
GPRAMA	GPRA Modernization Act
HHS	Department of Health and Human Services
HIE organization	health information exchange organization
HIPAA	Health Insurance Portability and Accountability Act

* This is an edited, reformatted and augmented version of The United States Government Accountability Office publication, GAO-14-242, dated March 2014.

HIT	health information technology
HITECH	Health Information Technology for Economic and Clinical Health Act
ONC	Office of the National Coordinator for Health Information Technology
REC	regional extension center
Recovery Act	American Recovery and Reinvestment Act of 2009
RFI	request for information
SNOMED CT	Systematized Nomenclature of Medicine Clinical Terms

WHY GAO DID THIS STUDY

The Health Information Technology for Economic and Clinical Health Act (HITECH) promotes the use of health information technology and identifies the importance of health information exchange. It provides incentive payments to promote the widespread adoption and meaningful use of EHR technology. To be a meaningful user, providers are to demonstrate, among other things, that their certified EHR technology can electronically exchange health information. GAO examined (1) the key challenges to the electronic exchange of health information, if any, that have been reported by providers and stakeholders, and HHS's ongoing efforts to address them, and (2) the extent to which HHS has planned future actions to address those key challenges. GAO reviewed HHS documentation; interviewed HHS officials; and interviewed providers— hospital officials and physicians—and relevant stakeholders about their experiences.

WHAT GAO RECOMMENDS

GAO recommends that CMS and ONC (1) develop and prioritize specific actions that HHS will take consistent with the principles in HHS's strategy to advance health information exchange, and (2) develop milestones with time frames for the actions to better gauge progress toward advancing exchange, with appropriate adjustments over time. In commenting on the draft report, HHS, including CMS and ONC, concurred with these recommendations.

What GAO Found

Providers and stakeholders GAO interviewed in four states with ongoing electronic health information exchange efforts cited key challenges to exchange, in particular, issues related to insufficient standards, concerns about how privacy rules can vary among states, difficulties in matching patients to their records, and costs associated with exchange. Officials from the Centers for Medicare & Medicaid Services (CMS) and the Office of the National Coordinator for Health Information Technology (ONC)—agencies within the Department of Health and Human Services (HHS)—noted that they have several ongoing programs and initiatives to help address some aspects of these key challenges, but concerns in these areas continue to exist. For example, several providers GAO interviewed said that they have difficulty exchanging certain types of health information due to insufficient health data standards. Although HHS has begun to address insufficiencies in standards through its Medicare and Medicaid Electronic Health Record (EHR) programs, such as through the introduction of new 2014 standards for certified EHR technology, it is unclear whether its efforts will lead to widespread improvements in electronic health information exchange. In addition, providers GAO interviewed reported challenges covering costs associated with electronic exchange, such as upfront costs associated with purchasing and implementing EHR systems. While HHS is working to address this challenge through various efforts, including a program that helps fund health information exchange organizations—organizations that provide support to facilitate the electronic exchange of health information—some providers told GAO they do not participate in these organizations because they see limited opportunities for exchanging information through them.

HHS, including CMS and ONC, developed and issued a strategy document in August 2013 that describes how it expects to advance electronic health information exchange. The strategy identifies principles intended to guide future actions to address the key challenges that providers and stakeholders have identified. However, the HHS strategy does not specify any such actions, how any actions should be prioritized, what milestones the actions need to achieve, or when these milestones need to be accomplished. GAO's prior work, consistent with the Government Performance and Results Act Modernization Act of 2010 (GPRAMA), sets forth several key elements of strategies that can guide agencies in planning and implementing an effective government program. As noted in GAO's prior work, elements such as specific actions, priorities, and milestones are desirable for evaluating progress, achieving results in specified time frames, and ensuring effective oversight and accountability. Determining specific actions and exchange-related milestones with specified time frames can help to ensure that the agencies' principles and future actions result in timely improvements in addressing the key challenges reported by providers and stakeholders; this is particularly important because planning for Stage 3 of the EHR programs, which focuses on improving outcomes, is expected to begin as soon as 2014. This information could also help CMS and ONC prioritize their future actions based on whether health information is being exchanged effectively among providers, in order to better achieve the EHR programs' ultimate goals of improving quality, efficiency, and patient safety.

* * *

March 24, 2014

Congressional Committees

The use of health information technology (HIT), such as electronic health record (EHR) systems, has the potential to allow health care providers and others to exchange health care information electronically, which is a key way that this technology could lead to improved health care quality and reduced costs. Health information exchange is especially important because the health care system is highly fragmented, with care and services provided in multiple settings, such as physician offices and hospitals, that may not be coordinated with each other.[1] Because of this fragmentation, providers may lack ready access to critical information needed to, for example, coordinate the care of patients to ensure they make the most-informed decisions on treatment options. Lack of care coordination can lead to inappropriate or duplicative tests and procedures that increase health care spending. Estimates of this spending increase range from $148 billion to $226 billion per year.[2]

To deliver coordinated care, a physician and other members of the care team must access and share health information from multiple settings. Providers may share clinical data using manual methods such as faxing paper records, but these methods can be time consuming and costly and are often unavailable at the point of care. In addition, data shared via manual methods are generally not structured or captured electronically to be stored in EHRs. Lacking the ability to receive and store structured data in their systems, providers may not be able to easily search for the information they need or electronically transmit the information effectively to another EHR without manual efforts. Electronic health information exchange has the potential to bring patient information directly from an EHR to the provider delivering care, regardless of where the care or services are delivered. Electronically exchanging information can facilitate care coordination and improve communication among providers, staff, and patients by making patient clinical information more readily available to providers. Electronically exchanging information is also important in new delivery system and payment models, such as accountable care organizations (ACO), because of the need for providers in different settings to have ready access to information needed to manage and coordinate care.[3]

The Health Information Technology for Economic and Clinical Health Act (HITECH), enacted as part of the American Recovery and Reinvestment Act of 2009 (Recovery Act), provided funding for various activities intended to promote the adoption and meaningful use of certified EHR technology.[4] HITECH identified the importance of the electronic exchange of health information by requiring it as a key element in the definition of meaningful use of certified EHR technology.[5] Specifically, in order to be a meaningful EHR user, providers are to demonstrate that their certified EHR technology is able to electronically exchange health information to improve the quality of health care, such as by promoting care coordination. As such, electronic exchange is of key importance to the Department of Health and Human Services' (HHS) Medicare and Medicaid EHR programs, which are intended to help increase the meaningful use of EHR technology and which are estimated to include total spending of $30 billion from 2011 through 2019.[6]

Research suggests that despite substantial growth in EHR adoption, electronic exchanges between providers have remained limited.[7] HITECH requires us to report on, among other things, its effect on the adoption of EHRs by providers.[8] We issued five reports on the EHR programs' implementation.[9] For example, in March 2014, we reported on the extent to which providers have met measures of meaningful use, including measures that involved the electronic exchange of health information, and noted that providers may face challenges meeting some of these measures under the EHR programs. As discussed with the committees of jurisdiction, this report addresses the electronic exchange of health information and serves as one of the series of reports we conducted to respond to the mandate. Specifically, this report examines (1) the key challenges to the electronic exchange of health information, if any, that have been reported by providers and stakeholders, and HHS's ongoing efforts to address these challenges, and (2) the extent to which

HHS has planned future actions to address the key challenges, if any, reported by providers and stakeholders.

To examine the key challenges to the electronic exchange of health information, if any, reported by providers and stakeholders, and HHS's ongoing efforts to address these challenges, we selected four states— Georgia, North Carolina, Minnesota, and Massachusetts—in which to interview selected providers and other relevant stakeholders to learn about the exchange of health information within their respective states.[10] We initially interviewed selected providers in Georgia, and then selected the additional states of North Carolina, Minnesota, and Massachusetts because they were mentioned during interviews with stakeholders and officials from HHS as having ongoing efforts related to health information exchange.[11] These three states also had an existing Pioneer ACO or a Beacon Community in which providers were likely to have some experience attempting to electronically exchange health information.[12] In each of the four selected states, we asked officials from the Regional Extension Centers (REC) and health information exchange organizations (HIE organization) to tell us about the exchange activities occurring in their state and to help us identify providers—individual physicians, hospitals, and health systems—to learn about their efforts to exchange health information.[13] We also conducted interviews with other relevant stakeholders that include the American Hospital Association (AHA), the American Medical Association, the College of Healthcare Information Management Executives (CHIME), and two commonly used EHR vendors for providers that attested to meaningful use in 2012. We conducted a total of 30 interviews with providers and stakeholders. Findings based on these interviews cannot be generalized to all providers.

In addition to interviewing providers and stakeholders about electronic exchange and the challenges of such exchange, we also reviewed additional sources to supplement our interviews, such as published literature and written information provided from stakeholders such as CHIME and AHA, including their responses to HHS's March 2013 request for information (RFI) about interoperability and health information exchange.[14] To provide context for the challenges reported by providers and stakeholders and to identify HHS's ongoing efforts to address them, we interviewed officials from the Centers for Medicare & Medicaid Services (CMS) and the Office of the National Coordinator for Health Information Technology (ONC) and reviewed documents related to current HHS efforts on health information exchange.

To examine the extent to which HHS has planned future actions to address the key challenges, if any, reported by providers and stakeholders, we interviewed officials from CMS and ONC who are responsible for overseeing and managing the EHR programs and other relevant programs and initiatives related to health information exchange. We asked them about the key challenges reported to us by the providers and stakeholders we interviewed as well as key challenges we identified from documents. We also reviewed documents related to ongoing and future HHS health information exchange actions, including strategy documents, policies, and presentations. In addition, we reviewed relevant requirements in our previous work on the elements of an effective strategy, [15] which is consistent with the Government Performance and Results Act (GPRA) of 1993,[16] as amended by the GPRA Modernization Act (GPRAMA) of 2010.[17] We compared HHS's documentation that delineates its planned steps for health information exchange to these requirements.

We conducted this performance audit from February 2013 through March 2014 in accordance with generally accepted government auditing standards. Those standards require that we plan and perform the audit to obtain sufficient, appropriate evidence to provide a reasonable basis for our findings and conclusions based on our audit objectives. We believe that the evidence obtained provides a reasonable basis for our findings and conclusions based on our audit objectives.

BACKGROUND

Electronic Health Information Exchange

Approaches to electronic health information exchange have expanded in recent years with the increased adoption of EHRs and growth of HIE organizations. For example, some providers can electronically exchange clinical information via interoperable EHR systems. In cases in which providers wish to exchange electronic health information but do not have interoperable systems, HIE organizations can serve as key facilitators of exchange by providing for data connections among stakeholders, including laboratories, public health departments, hospitals, and physicians. Specifically, the use of EHR technology and the use of HIE organizations can allow providers to request and receive information about patients from other providers' records, such as medication lists, laboratory results, or previous diagnoses and hospitalizations. For example, when a provider requests information, the HIE organization may be able to identify the sources of the requested data and initiate the electronic transmission that delivers the data from another provider's EHR in a format that can be accepted and processed by the receiving provider's EHR. Examples of exchange activities that can occur using EHR technology directly between providers or through an HIE organization are shown in figure 1.

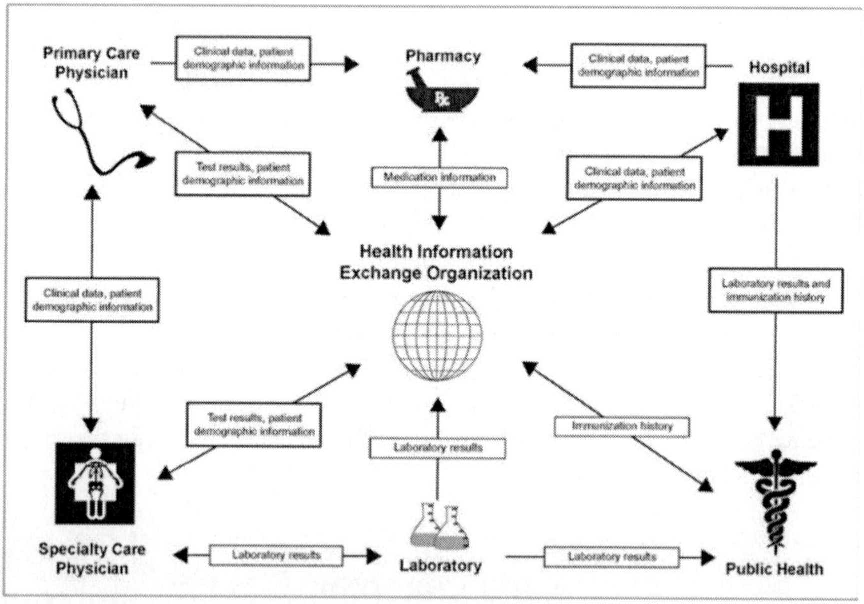

Source: GAO analysis (data); Art Explosion (clip art).

Figure 1. Examples of Health Information Exchange Using Electronic Health Record Technology.

According to an April 2012 article, exchanging EHR information with other entities can be significantly more difficult for a provider than using EHRs to manage health information within the provider's organization only—without exchanging the information with others.[18] Appendix I provides information about the extent to which providers are able to electronically exchange health information, as reported by providers and stakeholders we interviewed.

Medicare and Medicaid EHR Programs

HITECH provided funding for various activities, including the Medicare and Medicaid EHR programs. These programs are intended to help increase the meaningful use of EHR technology by providing incentive payments for, and later imposing penalties on, providers—that is, certain hospitals and health care professionals such as physicians—who participate in Medicare or Medicaid.[19] These programs are the largest of the activities, in terms of potential federal expenditures, funded by HITECH. Within HHS, CMS and ONC have developed the programs' requirements.[20]

CMS is responsible for administering the Medicare EHR program and overseeing and funding most of the Medicaid EHR program, which is administered by the states and U.S. insular areas.[21] For both EHR programs, CMS established specific requirements under three progressive stages of meaningful use that providers must meet to qualify for incentive payments.[22] As the programs progress through these stages, more requirements will be added:

- Stage 1, which began in 2011, set the basic functionalities EHRs must include, such as capturing data electronically and providing patients with electronic copies of health information.[23] CMS and ONC indicated that Stage 1 allowed providers to test the capability of their EHRs to electronically exchange health information.
- Stage 2, which began in 2014, added requirements such as increased health information exchange between providers to improve care coordination for patients. For example, Stage 2 will require hospitals and professionals to provide an electronic summary of care document for each transition of care or referral to another provider, whereas in Stage 1 this measure was optional.[24]
- Stage 3, which is scheduled to go into effect in 2017, will continue to expand on meaningful use to improve health care outcomes and the exchange of health information, according to CMS and ONC. The requirements for this stage have not yet been developed.

ONC is responsible for identifying health data standards and technical specifications for EHR technology and establishing and overseeing the certification of EHR technology.[25] As part of the EHR programs, providers must report annually on certain mandatory meaningful use measures and on additional measures that they may choose from a menu of measures. Appendix II describes those Stage 1 and Stage 2 meaningful use measures that CMS and ONC reported as specifically relating to health information exchange.

Challenges Are Reported Related to Standards, Privacy, Patient Matching, and Costs of Electronic Exchange

Providers and stakeholders we interviewed cited key challenges to electronic health information exchange; in particular, they cited issues related to insufficient standards, concerns about how privacy rules can vary among states, difficulties in matching patients to their records, and costs associated with electronic health information exchange. CMS and ONC officials noted that they have several ongoing programs and initiatives to help address some aspects of these key challenges, but concerns in these areas continue to exist.

Reported insufficiencies in standards for electronic health information exchange. While standards for electronically exchanging information within the EHR programs exist, providers reported that standards may not be sufficient in some areas. Information that is electronically exchanged from one provider to another must adhere to the same standards in order to be interpreted and used in EHRs, thereby permitting interoperability. Several providers stated that they often have difficulty exchanging certain types of health information with other providers that have a different EHR system due to a lack of sufficient standards to support exchange.

One area for which providers told us standards were insufficient relates to standards for allergies. Specifically, one provider noted that there are not sufficient standards to define allergic reactions, and another provider explained that some EHR systems classify an allergic reaction as a side effect, while other EHR systems classify the same reaction as an allergy. Such differences can cause confusion when health information is exchanged among providers because providers who receive information may have difficulty locating or using information on allergies if their EHR systems classify the information differently than the EHR systems of the providers who sent the information. Similarly, an article from the *Journal of the American Medical Informatics Association* stated that the proper terminology for encoding patients' allergies is complex and that some gaps still exist across existing standards.[26]

HHS has begun to address insufficiencies in standards through the EHR programs. In order to participate in the programs, providers must use EHR technology that has been certified by HHS to meet certain criteria. Specifically, the standards and certification criteria identify certain vocabularies and structured formats that must be included in certified EHR technology that providers use when exchanging health information.[27] HHS has issued a new edition of the standards and certification criteria that takes effect in 2014. Providers are required to use EHR technology certified to these standards beginning in 2014, regardless of whether they participated in the EHR programs in earlier years. Compared to the previous 2011 edition, the 2014 edition includes more certification criteria and specifies certain standards to support exchange, such as standards for the transmission of health information and a summary of care record standard that providers must use to participate in the EHR programs. For example, the standards require certified EHR technology to be able to transmit patient care summaries using a structured format, referred to as a continuity of care document (CCD), which allows providers to record health information using the same template.[28] In addition, in order to standardize the transmittal of health information, ONC has developed the Direct Protocol, which defines a standard format that providers can use to send secure health messages from one entity to another.[29] HHS expects that providers using the 2014 edition will have greater ability to exchange information.[30]

Although progress has been made, as represented by the 2014 edition of the standards and certification criteria, concerns regarding standards remain. First, while the 2014 edition certification standards may lead to a greater ability to exchange information and HHS has tested the implementation of the standards among certain providers, HHS officials told us that the extent to which the standards will lead to widespread improvements in electronic health information exchange will remain unclear until a larger number of providers begin using technology that is certified to the standards. Second, some concerns regarding standards were not addressed through the 2014 edition, and several providers we interviewed said there is a need for standards that would allow all certified EHR technology to be interoperable so all types of health information could be electronically exchanged across providers. In addition, the AHA, in its response to HHS's March 2013 RFI, stated that the 2014 edition does not require certified EHRs to support a standard to facilitate more advanced exchange than is supported by the Direct Protocol. The AHA noted that it is appropriate to require certified EHRs to support both the Direct Protocol and other standards that would allow for more robust exchange so providers can choose which standard is appropriate for their needs when exchanging health information. Third, some providers suggested that there is a need for standards that enable providers to electronically exchange more detailed clinical information, such as patient narratives, than what is included in a CCD.[31] Fourth, one provider we interviewed noted that standards regarding allergies were insufficient and that RxNorm and the Systematized Nomenclature of Medicine Clinical Terms

(SNOMED CT) should be expanded for nonmedication allergies and allergic reactions.[32] Fifth, several providers and stakeholders commented that the Direct Protocol allows for limited exchange, such as exchanging a secure email message, rather than enabling certain other functionalities, such as the ability to query another EHR system.[33]

Reported variation in state privacy rules and lack of clarity about requirements. Some providers noted that exchanging health information with providers in other states can be difficult due to their limited understanding of variations in privacy rules from state to state. Some providers also noted that exchange can be especially difficult in cases when providers are located close to state borders and therefore serve patients from another state. Providers that are covered by the Health Insurance Portability and Accountability Act (HIPAA) of 1996 must adhere to federal privacy rules and can also be subject to state privacy rules.[34] These state rules can be more stringent than HIPAA requirements or standards.

To address privacy issues related to electronic health information exchange, ONC officials have several ongoing efforts. For example, ONC has issued high-level guidance for providers on how to ensure the privacy and security of health information covering a wide range of topics related to meaningful use and the HIPAA Privacy and Security Rules, among other things. Regarding state privacy laws, this guidance suggests that providers seek information from state agencies, RECs, and professional associations to understand how state laws affect the sharing of patient health information. In addition, ONC began the Data Segmentation for Privacy Initiative to develop and pilot test standards for managing patient consents and data segmentation.[35] As part of this initiative, ONC released an implementation guide for consent management and data segmentation in the summer of 2012, and the agency is currently pilot testing this guide. In addition, ONC's state HIE organization program is currently receiving reports from states on how they are implementing their state's privacy rules. Officials expect to receive the information from states by March 2014. ONC officials are hopeful that these efforts will help address privacy concerns and, as a result, facilitate exchange efforts for providers.

Although ONC is working on privacy issues, some providers we spoke with reported that lack of clarity in state privacy laws is one reason that they have experienced difficulty exchanging health information with providers in other states. They found it difficult to ensure they were compliant with state laws when exchanging certain personal health information with providers in another state. For example, some providers in Minnesota and Massachusetts noted that some state laws have stringent requirements related to sharing health information related to mental health, or human immunodeficiency virus or other sexually transmitted infections. In addition, some providers told us that different providers in their state have different interpretations regarding how frequently they must obtain consent from the patient, as required under the state privacy rule, for the exchange of patients' health information. For example, some providers may interpret the state privacy rule to mean that every time a patient's health information is exchanged with another provider they have to obtain consent. Other providers in the same state may interpret the state privacy rule to mean that they have to obtain consent only once.

In addition to the privacy challenges identified by providers, stakeholders responding to HHS's March 2013 RFI also identified privacy as a challenge related to health information exchange, and noted that additional training for providers on varying state privacy laws is needed to address this challenge. Stakeholders also suggested that HHS could focus more resources on consent policies and recommended that HHS undertake additional work to facilitate (1) electronically obtaining patient consent for disclosing health information, and (2) communicating that consent along with the related health information.

Reported difficulty of accurately matching patients to their health records. Some providers we interviewed reported that they do not have an accurate and efficient way to match patients to their records when exchanging health information. Multiple providers and stakeholders cited situations in which several of their patients are listed with the same name and birth year, and live in the same area. Two of these providers reported that patients can be matched to the wrong set of records, and that providers often need to manually match records, which is time-consuming. Some stakeholders also noted similar problems, including safety concerns from incorrect patient matching.

HHS programs or initiatives to address patient matching issues related to health information exchange include both a patient matching project and efforts by two federal advisory committees. According to ONC officials, planning for the Patient Matching Initiative was begun by the State Health Information Exchange Cooperative Agreement Program in July 2013, and the project launched publicly in September 2013. The goals of the initiative are to (1) improve patient matching based on an assessment of current approaches used by selected stakeholders, (2) identify key attributes and algorithms for matching patients to their records, and (3) define processes or best practices to support the identified key attributes. The first phase of the initiative was completed in February 2014 with the release of a report containing patient matching recommendations for possible inclusion in Stage 3 of the EHR programs and the 2015 edition of the standards and certification criteria.[36] The two federal advisory committees established under HITECH, the HIT Policy Committee and the HIT Standards Committee, made recommendations to HHS in 2011 that relate to patient matching.[37] The HIT Policy Committee recommended standardized formats for demographic data fields, internally evaluating matching accuracy, accountability, developing, promoting and disseminating best practices, and supporting the role of the patient. The HIT Standards Committee made four recommendations on patient matching covering patient attributes that could be used, data quality issues, formats for data elements, and the data that could be returned from a match request. According to ONC officials, as of July 2013 ONC had efforts under way to respond to these recommendations, under the Patient Matching Initiative, in coordination with the committees. For example, to address one recommendation related to developing, promoting, and disseminating best practices, ONC officials said that they plan to determine which approaches to patient matching work best and develop guidance to help organizations implement such steps.

Although HHS has ongoing efforts to address the patient matching challenge, several providers and stakeholders commented that more work needs to be done on this issue. Some providers we interviewed use different methodologies, such as algorithms that make use of multiple patient attributes for identifying patients. However, providers told us that they still have challenges matching patients to their records. Several providers and stakeholders have stated that there should be a national patient identifier for matching patients to their records.[38] Some stakeholders who responded to HHS's March 2013 RFI stated that HHS has an opportunity to reduce the potential risks of engaging in exchange by focusing more resources on patient matching.

Reported challenges with cost of exchanging health information. Providers we interviewed reported challenges covering costs associated with health information exchange, including upfront costs associated with purchasing and implementing EHR systems, fees for participation in state or local HIE organizations, and per-transaction fees for exchanging health information charged by some vendors or HIE organizations. Several providers said that they must invest in additional capabilities such as establishing interfaces for exchange with laboratories or other entities such as HIE organizations. For example, many providers told us that the cost of developing, implementing, and maintaining interfaces with others to exchange health information is a significant barrier. One provider and several officials estimated various amounts between $50,000 and $80,000 that providers spend to establish data exchange interfaces. Other stakeholders we interviewed or who responded to HHS's March 2013 RFI also identified costs associated with participation in HIE organizations and maintaining EHR systems as a challenge for providers.

To address costs of exchanging health information, ONC's State Health Information Exchange Cooperative Agreement Program has provided funding to HIE organizations.[39] Agency officials stated that by funding HIE organizations, a relatively low cost option can be made available for providers to use to exchange health information. However, ONC officials said that this program is scheduled to end in March 2014.[40] In addition, several providers we interviewed told us that for them the benefits to them of joining an HIE organization often do not exceed the costs, in some cases because few providers have joined their state or regional HIE organizations, resulting in limited opportunities to exchange health information. Some providers told us they do not participate in HIE organizations because they exchange information in other ways that they believe are more efficient, such as exchanging directly with other providers that use the same EHR system from the same vendor. One study noted that most health care providers, including over 65 percent of hospitals and 90 percent of physician practices, were not participating in HIE organizations.[41]

HHS payments to providers under the EHR programs can help support the cost of exchange, but providers can participate in the programs without routinely exchanging information electronically that could lead to improved care. While some of the meaningful use requirements for Stage 1 and Stage 2 help to facilitate the exchange of health information, they require exchange only under certain circumstances. (See app. II for more information.) For example, one part of the requirement to provide a summary care document for each transition of care or referral in Stage 2 compels providers to complete either (1) one successful electronic exchange of a summary of care record with a recipient using technology designed by an EHR developer other than the sender's, or (2) one successful test with CMS's test EHR during the reporting period.[42] One stakeholder we spoke with explained that for this part of the requirement some providers just complete one successful test with CMS's test EHR and do not routinely demonstrate exchanging health information electronically with other EHR systems. HHS officials stated that Stage 2 is an incremental step toward advancing exchange, and that providers generally do not yet have the technology to enable greater exchange.

HHS Developed an Electronic Health Information Exchange Strategy That Includes Principles to Address Key Challenges but Lacks Specific Prioritized Actions and Milestones

HHS, including CMS and ONC, developed and issued a strategy document in August 2013 that describes how it expects to advance electronic health information exchange, with principles to guide future actions in three broad areas—accelerating health information exchange, advancing standards and interoperability, and patient engagement.[43] Examples of principles in the strategy include (1) working with multiple stakeholders to develop standards and facilitating the adoption and use of standards among federal agencies; (2) supporting the privacy, security, and integrity of patient health information across health information exchange activities; (3) seeking to enable a patient's health information to be available wherever the patient accesses care, to support patient-centered care delivery; and (4) supporting exchange through state-led efforts to reduce costs to providers. (See app. III for a complete list of principles.) According to the strategy, these principles have the potential to address the key health information challenges identified by providers and stakeholders we interviewed, which relate to standards, patients' privacy, matching patients with data, and costs.

While HHS officials intend these principles to lead to future actions that have the potential to address key challenges, the HHS strategy does not specify any such actions, how any actions should be prioritized, what milestones the actions need to achieve, or when milestones need to be accomplished. Our previous work, consistent with GPRAMA, sets forth several key elements of strategies that can guide agencies in planning and implementing an effective government program. [44] As noted in our prior work, elements such as specific actions, priorities, and milestones are desirable for evaluating progress, achieving results in specific time frames, and ensuring effective oversight and accountability. These elements can also be used to gauge progress when implementing programs and to determine whether adjustments need to be made in order to maintain progress within given time frames.[45] Below are examples of how the lack of these elements affects the HHS strategy.

- *Specific Actions.* While the strategy mentions that HHS seeks to enable a patient's health information to be available wherever the patient accesses care, it does not indicate specific actions that HHS will take to implement that principle or how those actions would overcome exchange-related challenges. Including specific actions could enhance the strategy's usefulness for helping to make program management decisions.
- *Prioritized Actions.* While the HHS strategy states that HHS will continue to evaluate short- and long-term steps to advance exchange, it does not clearly delineate how future actions related to the principles should be prioritized. Prioritizing actions can help HHS ensure that the most appropriate activities are completed first, to more efficiently achieve the goal of advancing exchange.
- *Milestones.* The HHS strategy does not provide milestones with specific time frames to help the agencies gauge their progress in advancing exchange. Exchange-related milestones with specified time frames could be particularly useful because they could provide a framework for determining whether any actions HHS intends to take could help lead to progress in addressing the challenges providers face related to exchange. Milestones with time frames could also set realistic expectations so stakeholders can anticipate when they can expect to see actions to advance exchange.

CMS and ONC officials acknowledged the importance of providers being able to exchange health information effectively by Stage 3 of the EHR programs to allow for improved outcomes such as quality, efficiency, and patient safety. Determining specific, prioritized actions and exchange-related milestones with specified time frames can help to ensure that the agencies' principles and future actions result in timely improvements in addressing the key exchange-related challenges reported by providers and stakeholders, which are particularly important because planning for Stage 3 is expected to begin as soon as 2014. This information could also help HHS prioritize its future actions based on whether health information is being exchanged effectively among providers, in order to better achieve the EHR programs' ultimate goals of improving quality, efficiency, and patient safety.

Conclusion

HHS and providers have made some progress toward addressing challenges reported by providers and others related to the electronic exchange of health information, but these challenges are complex and difficult to address and are likely to continue to persist. Some of HHS's most important efforts, such as designing the 2014 edition of the standards and certification criteria to include an increased exchange capability in EHR systems, may lead to greater exchange over the next year. In addition, exchange may increase as providers modify their systems to meet more stringent exchange-related requirements in Stage 2 of the EHR programs. However, a number of remaining challenges make these outcomes uncertain.

HHS has both ongoing programs and future plans to address concerns about exchange, but it is not always clear how HHS will effectively prioritize and implement its potential responses to the challenges of exchange. Specifically, the HHS strategy to advance electronic health information exchange does not identify specific actions that CMS and ONC expect will lead to increased exchange, prioritize these actions, or include milestones for gauging progress over time. Guidance on planning and implementing effective strategies highlights the importance of key elements, such as specific, prioritized actions and milestones for gauging progress. These elements could help the agencies make future adjustments based on the effectiveness of their efforts. Exchange is especially important because of its potential to help improve coordination of care within the fragmented health care system. According to CMS and ONC officials, ensuring progress in providers' ability to electronically exchange information is critical for the effective implementation of the EHR programs. Without a sufficient focus on exchange—including specific, prioritized actions with milestones and time frames—CMS and ONC run the risk that the desired outcomes of the EHR programs of improved quality, efficiency, and patient safety will be compromised.

Recommendations for Executive Action

To address challenges that affect the ability of providers to electronically exchange health information, we recommend that the Secretary of Health and Human Services direct CMS and ONC to take the following two actions:

- develop and prioritize specific actions that HHS will take consistent with the principles in HHS's strategy to advance health information exchange; and
- develop milestones with time frames for the actions to better gauge progress toward advancing exchange, with appropriate adjustments over time.

AGENCY COMMENTS

We provided a draft of this report to HHS for comment. HHS concurred with our recommendations. For the first recommendation, HHS (including CMS and ONC) stated that it has begun to develop and prioritize specific action items, consistent with the principles in its strategy to advance health information exchange, and that it has begun to take action on some of the prioritized items. For the second recommendation, HHS (including CMS and ONC) stated that it has begun developing milestones with time frames for the actions to better gauge progress toward advancing exchange. In general, HHS's comments also reiterated that the electronic exchange of health information is a key element of meaningful use and ultimately will be critical for the success of health care delivery system reforms under the Patient Protection and Affordable Care Act. HHS also stated that it has begun to take definitive steps to accelerate exchange through policy guidance, grant funding to states, and development of standards and certification, such as collaborating with private sector organizations that develop health IT standards to fill key gaps in standards to better support information exchange during transitions in care and when coordinating care across providers. Additionally, HHS provided technical comments, which we incorporated as appropriate.

Linda T. Kohn
Director,
Health Care

APPENDIX I: INFORMATION REPORTED BY PROVIDERS ON THE ELECTRONIC EXCHANGE OF HEALTH INFORMATION AND ITS RELATED BENEFITS

This appendix provides additional information reported from providers we spoke with about health information exchange and its related benefits. We conducted a total of 25 interviews with providers and stakeholders, such as regional extension centers (REC) and health information exchange organizations (HIE organization), in four states—Georgia, Massachusetts, Minnesota, and North Carolina. We interviewed staff from at least two hospitals or health systems and at least one physician office or group practice in each state. We selected the four states because they were mentioned during interviews with officials from HHS and relevant stakeholders as having ongoing efforts related to health information exchange. We asked interviewees about what types of patient health information providers are currently able to electronically exchange, the methods used to exchange such information, and the benefits providers have realized or foresee from such exchange.

Providers we interviewed reported that the most critical types of health information that they need to be able to electronically exchange include patient allergy information, medication lists, and problem lists. However, providers generally reported being able to electronically exchange only specific types of health information at this time, including lab orders and results, immunization and prescription information, and certain clinical documents. For example,

- Almost all the providers we interviewed reported some exchange of lab information. In most cases, such exchanges involved both the submission of lab orders and the receipt of lab results via interfaces designed for exchange between providers and labs or through their electronic health record (EHR) system. While these exchanges were reported to generally occur between providers and laboratories outside their organizations, two providers noted that such capabilities were still limited to sharing lab information with others in the same health system.
- Some providers also reported electronically exchanging some information with state public health departments, generally immunization data and notification of certain infectious diseases. They said that these electronic exchanges were generally limited to

submissions to the departments and did not include receipt of data from these departments.

- Several of the providers we interviewed said they engaged in e-prescribing activities, which in some instances included both the submission of electronic prescriptions to pharmacies and the receipt of medication information from pharmacies. However, some providers noted that such exchanges could take place only if the pharmacy had a compatible e-prescribing system that could electronically receive prescription information from the provider's EHR system. In the absence of compatible systems, faxes were used.
- Several providers we interviewed also noted that they could exchange continuity of care documents (CCD) with other providers in their organization, although the exchange of this type of information varied among the providers we interviewed.[1] Several providers said they could exchange CCDs within their health system, whereas other providers said they could exchange this information only with providers using the same EHR vendor.

Providers in all four states and stakeholders that we interviewed reported that, at this time, methods used to electronically exchange health information are limited to use within health systems, use between certain EHR systems, or use of the Direct Protocol. 2 For example,

- In Georgia, REC officials and the four providers we spoke with told us that electronic exchange is generally occurring only within health systems and among those affiliated providers that work in the health systems. Some providers noted that they could electronically exchange lab orders and results outside their organizations, but one provider noted that even this information was still exchanged electronically only within its hospital.
- Providers in Minnesota, Massachusetts, and North Carolina reported that they used the same EHR system from the same vendor and were able to electronically exchange all patient clinical information with any other entity using that vendor via an interoperability feature.[3]
  According to these providers, this interoperability feature provides a mechanism for them to electronically exchange all types of clinical information about their patients.

- A community-based hospital in Minnesota reported using a different EHR system than was used by the other, larger health systems in the community it shared information with. This provider reported relying on the Direct Protocol to electronically exchange some limited health information with other providers in the region. A provider in Massachusetts noted that it was building web-based "view portals" to allow other providers outside its health system to view health information electronically in order to help coordinate patient care.

Providers that participated in an HIE organization reported being able to electronically exchange health information with other providers. Others have opted to electronically exchange information using their EHR technology rather than an HIE organization, even if one was available.

- In Massachusetts, some providers told us that they are able to directly connect to the state's HIE organization in order to electronically exchange health information, such as CCDs. However, not all providers in the state are electronically exchanging information at this time. A Massachusetts law calls for the creation and maintenance of a state HIE organization that allows providers in all health care settings to exchange patient health information with other providers by the end of 2016.[4]
- Some providers we spoke with in Minnesota said they had no plans to join any of the HIE organizations available in the state at this time due to the limited benefits they would realize from participating, and would instead continue to rely on their EHR technology to electronically exchange health information with other providers that use the same vendor. Some providers noted that without a sufficient number of other providers participating in an HIE organization, it would be of limited value.
- Several Georgia and North Carolina providers reported that the availability of an HIE organization could help facilitate electronic exchange among providers. Entities in both states are establishing regional HIE organizations that will ultimately connect to one another via a statewide HIE organization. Providers in both states said they expected that the HIE organizations, once established, would facilitate broader electronic exchange of health information throughout the state.

Although providers we interviewed described certain circumstances when they could electronically exchange health information, they indicated that they would like to expand the electronic exchange of health information and cited a variety of benefits related to such electronic exchange. For example, some providers noted that electronic exchange can

- provide access to critical information needed when administering medical care, thus improving care quality and reducing duplicative testing;
- improve access to information related to a patient's health history, including medication histories and previous diagnoses;
- result in more timely access to information, which is particularly helpful in emergency departments; and
- reduce labor-intensive efforts to send and receive health information in paper form, such as a printed document, or conduct public health reporting activities.

APPENDIX II: STAGE 1 AND STAGE 2 MEANINGFUL USE MEASURES RELATED TO ELECTRONIC HEALTH INFORMATION EXCHANGE

This appendix provides information on the Stage 1 and Stage 2 meaningful use measures related to electronic health information exchange, according to officials from the Centers for Medicare & Medicaid Services (CMS) and the Office of the National Coordinator for Health Information Technology (ONC). According to these officials, Stage 2, which began in 2014, provides additional requirements related to the exchange of health information. For example, some meaningful use measures related to health information exchange that providers could select from a menu of optional measures in Stage 1 are mandatory for Stage 2. In addition, some Stage 2 measures are new. For example, the measure "provide structured electronic lab results to ambulatory providers" is a new measure for hospitals in Stage 2. See table 1 for more information.

Table 1. Meaningful Use Measures Related to Electronic Health Information Exchange According to the Centers for Medicare & Medicaid Services (CMS) and the Office of the National Coordinator for Health Information Technology (ONC), Stage 1 and Stage 2

	Hospitals		*Professionals*	
Meaningful use measure related to electronic health information exchange	*Stage 1*	*Stage 2*	*Stage 1*	*Stage 2*
Generate and transmit permissible prescriptions electronically: For hospitals for Stage 2, generate, transmit, and check each prescription for the existence of a relevant drug formulary for more than 10 percent of hospital discharge prescriptions; for professionals, generate and transmit more than 40 percent (for Stage 1) or more than 50 percent (for Stage 2) of permissible prescriptions electronically and for Stage 2 also check each prescription for the existence of a relevant formulary			•	•
Provide patients with their health information electronically: For Stage 1: provide information (for hospitals and professionals, provide diagnostic test results, problem list, medication lists, and medication allergies, and for hospitals also provide discharge summary and procedures) within 3 business days to more than 50 percent of patients who requested to receive that information electronically. For Stage 2: provide more than 50 percent of patients online access to their health information within 36 hours of discharge (for hospitals) or	•[a]	•	•[a]	•

	Hospitals		*Professionals*	
Meaningful use measure related to electronic health information exchange	*Stage 1*	*Stage 2*	*Stage 1*	*Stage 2*
4 days (for professionals); more than 5 percent of patients view, download, or transmit their health information to a third party				
For hospitals, provide patients with electronic copy of discharge instructions at the time of discharge, upon request; for professionals, provide patients with clinical summaries for each office visit: For hospitals, provide information for more than 50 percent of patients who requested that information; for professionals, provide information for more than 50 percent of visits within 3 business days for Stage 1 or 1 business day for Stage 2	●	[b]	●[c]	●
Exchange key clinical information electronically: Perform at least one test of electronic health record technology's capacity to exchange key clinical information	●[d]		●[d]	
Incorporate clinical lab-test results into electronic health records as structured data: Incorporate into the electronic health record technology more than 40 percent (for Stage 1) or 55 percent (for Stage 2) of the clinical lab test results ordered whose results are positive, negative, or in numerical format	○[e]	●[e]	○[e]	●[e]
Perform medication reconciliation for patients received from another setting of care or provider of care: Perform for more than 50 percent of	○[c]	●[c]	○[c]	●[c]

Table 1. (Continued)

	Hospitals		*Professionals*	
Meaningful use measure related to electronic health information exchange	*Stage 1*	*Stage 2*	*Stage 1*	*Stage 2*
transitions of care				
Provide summary of care document for each transition of care or referral: For Stage 1 and Stage 2, provide for more than 50 percent of transitions of care and referrals; for Stage 2 also (a) provide for more than 10 percent of transitions of care and referrals either electronically transmitted using certified electronic health record technology or through an exchange with a Nationwide Health Information Network Exchange participant or in a way that is consistent with the Nationwide Health Information Networkfand (b) conduct one or more successful electronic exchanges of a summary of care document with a recipient with electronic health record technology designed by a different developer than the sender's or conduct one or more successful tests with the CMS-designated test electronic health record	○	●	○	●
Submit electronic data to immunization registries or immunization information systems: For Stage 1, perform at least one test of electronic health record technology's capacity to submit data to immunization registries and, if test is successful, institute regular	○	●	○	●

	Hospitals		*Professionals*	
Meaningful use measure related to electronic health information exchange	*Stage 1*	*Stage 2*	*Stage 1*	*Stage 2*
reporting; for Stage 2, demonstrate successful ongoing submission of data to immunization registries				
Submit electronic syndromic surveillance data to public health agencies: For Stage 1, perform at least one test of electronic health record technology's capacity to submit data to public health agencies and, if test is successful, institute regular reporting; for Stage 2, demonstrate successful ongoing submission of data to public health agencies	○	●	○	○
Submit electronic data on reportable lab results to public health agencies: For Stage 1, perform at least one test of electronic health record technology's capacity to submit data (as required by state or local law) to public health agencies and, if test is successful, institute regular reporting; for Stage 2, demonstrate successful ongoing submission of data (as required by state or local law) to public health agencies	○	●		
Use secure electronic messaging to communicate with patients: More than 5 percent of patients sent the professional a secure message				●
Provide patients with timely electronic access to their health information: Provide electronic access to health information (including lab results, problem list,			○[g]	[b]

Table 1. (Continued)

	Hospitals		*Professionals*	
Meaningful use measure related to electronic health information exchange	*Stage 1*	*Stage 2*	*Stage 1*	*Stage 2*
medication lists, and allergies) to at least 10 percent of patients within 4 business days				
Ensure that imaging results and accompanying information are accessible through certified electronic health record technology: Make more than 10 percent of all tests with one or more images accessible through certified electronic health record technology		○		○
Demonstrate capability to identify and report cancer cases to public health central cancer registry: Demonstrate successful ongoing submission of cancer case information from certified electronic health record technology to a public health central cancer registry				○
Demonstrate capability to identify and report specific cases to a specialized registry: Demonstrate successful ongoing submission of specific case information from certified electronic health record technology to a specialized registry other than a cancer registry				○
Provide structured electronic lab results to ambulatory providers: Send structured electronic clinical lab results to the ordering provider for more than 20 percent of electronic lab orders		○		

Source: GAO analysis of guidance from the Centers for Medicare & Medicaid Services (CMS) and of information obtained from officials from CMS and the Office of the National Coordinator for Health Information Technology (ONC).

Note: Mandatory measures are indicated by a filled circle (●), and optional measures are indicated by an open circle (○).

[a] Beginning in 2014, the Stage 2 criteria apply for Stage 1 with the exception that there is no requirement that patients view, download, or transmit their health information.

[b] For Stage 2, this measure was incorporated into the "provide patients with their health information electronically" measure.

[c] ONC did not indicate that this measure is related to health information exchange.

[d] This requirement was eliminated from the Stage 1 requirements beginning in 2013.

[e] While CMS officials did not indicate that this measure is related to the actual transfer of health information between entities, they did explain that this measure helps enable exchange by allowing information to be structured in such a way that when it is transferred it is usable by the recipient. CMS officials also stated that various other meaningful use measures (not included in this table) fulfill this purpose.

[f] The Nationwide Health Information Network, funded by ONC, provides a set of standards, services, and policies that enable the secure exchange of health information over the Internet.

[g] This requirement was eliminated from the Stage 1 requirements beginning in 2014.

Appendix III: CMS and ONC Principles to Facilitate Health Information Exchange

This appendix provides information on the principles that the Centers for Medicare & Medicaid Services (CMS) and the Office of the National Coordinator for Health Information Technology (ONC) plan to use to guide their future actions to facilitate health information exchange. These principles are outlined in a strategy that the agencies released in August 2013 to describe how they expect the principles to lead to future actions that have the potential to address the key challenges providers and stakeholders have identified relative to electronic health information exchange in four areas—standards, patients' privacy, matching patients with data, and costs.[1] The strategy includes principles under three broad categories—accelerating health information exchange, advancing standards and interoperability, and patient engagement. See table 2 for more information.

Table 2. The Centers for Medicare & Medicaid Services (CMS) and the Office of the National Coordinator for Health Information Technology (ONC) Principles Related to Health Information Exchange

CMS and ONC Categories	CMS and ONC Principles
Accelerating Health Information Exchange	Seek to ensure that all new regulations and guidance on existing programs enable a patient's health information to follow them wherever they access care to support patient-centered care delivery.
	Implement policies that encourage health information exchange incrementally and couldevolve from incentive and reward structures to ultimately considering health information exchange a standard business practice for providers.
	Enable health information exchange where possible in support of state-led delivery and payment reform through federal and state partnerships.
	Encourage interoperability across states' electronic information infrastructures, includingMedicaid and State Survey Agencies and other Department of Health and Human Services (HHS)–funded enterprise systems.
	Collaborate with other departments in the federal government to facilitate the adoption and use of HHS health information technology (HIT) standards and interoperability requirements by those departments and their constituents.
	Educate consumers from diverse cultural and socioeconomic backgrounds on health information exchange and what it means for them.
	Support the privacy, security, and integrity of patient health information across all of its health information exchange acceleration activities.
Advancing Standards and Interoperability	Advance multi-stakeholder development of standards through the Standards and Interoperability Framework and coordination with standards development organizations such as Health Level 7 International[a]
	Accelerate interoperability through adoption of HIT standards through a variety of policies and programs, informed by advice from the HIT Policy Committee, the HIT Standards Committee, and the National Committee on

CMS and ONC Categories	CMS and ONC Principles
	Vital and Health Statistics.
	Align HIT standards for quality measurement and improvement across Medicare and Medicaid programs when appropriate.
	Accelerate alignment and implementation of electronic clinical quality measures, electronic decision support interventions, and electronic reporting mechanisms.
	Develop standards and policies to enable electronic management of consent and health information exchange among providers treating patients with sensitive health data such as those with behavioral health conditions or HIV.
	Strengthen data provenance to enhance providers' confidence in the original source of the data they receive.
Patient engagement	Support appropriate patient access to their health information.
	Support appropriate access to a patient's health information by family care givers.
	Make HHS standardized data available to patients wherever possible.

Source: GAO analysis of HHS data.

[a]Health Level 7 International is an organization that develops standards for exchanging electronic health information. These standards define how information is packaged and communicated from one entity to another, setting the language, structure, and data types required for integration between systems.

End Notes

[1] We use the term health information exchange to refer to the sharing of health information among organizations. The term is also used elsewhere to refer to a stakeholder organization that provides services to enable the electronic sharing of health-related information among providers and other entities, such as public health departments; we refer to such an organization as a health information exchange organization (HIE organization).

[2] D. Berwick and A. Hackbarth, "Eliminating Waste in U.S. Health Care," Journal of the American Medical Association, vol. 307, no. 14 (2012).

[3] An ACO is a group of providers and suppliers of services, such as hospitals and physicians, that work together to coordinate care for the patients they serve.

[4] HITECH was enacted as title XIII of division A and title IV of division B of the Recovery Act. Pub. L. No. 111-5, div. A, tit. XIII, 123 Stat. 115, 226-279 and div. B, tit. IV, 123 Stat. 115, 467-496 (2009).

To be certified, EHR technology must meet certain criteria established by HHS's Office of the National Coordinator for Health Information Technology that describe minimum related performance standards and implementation specifications. Certified EHR technology helps assure purchasers and other users that an EHR offers a minimum level of technological capability, functionality, and security.

[5] HITECH defined a meaningful EHR user as one who, in addition to using certified technology to electronically exchange health information, demonstrates to the satisfaction of the Secretary of Health and Human Services that (1) the technology is certified and being used in a meaningful manner, and (2) the certified technology is used to submit information on clinical quality measures and other measures in a form and manner specified by the Secretary. See Pub. L. No. 111-5, § 4101(a), 123 Stat. 467-472.

[6] Congressional Budget Office, "Health Information Technology for Economic and Clinical Health Act" (Washington, D.C.: Jan. 21, 2009).

[7] C. DesRoches et al., "Adoption of Electronic Health Records Grows Rapidly, but Fewer Than Half of US Hospitals Had at Least a Basic System in 2012," Health Affairs, vol. 32, no. 8 (2013); and M. Furukawa et al., "Hospital Electronic Health Information Exchange Grew Substantially In 2008-12," Health Affairs, vol. 32, no. 8 (2013).

[8] See Pub. L. No. 111-5, § 13424(e), 123 Stat. 278-279.

[9] GAO, Electronic Health Records: First Year of CMS's Incentive Programs Shows Opportunities to Improve Processes to Verify Providers Met Requirements, GAO-12-481 (Washington, D.C.: Apr. 30, 2012); Electronic Health Records: Number and Characteristics of Providers Awarded Medicare Incentive Payments for 2011, GAO-12-778R (Washington, D.C.: July 26, 2012); Electronic Health Records: Number and Characteristics of Providers Awarded Medicaid Incentive Payments for 2011, GAO-13-146R (Washington, D.C.: Dec. 13, 2012); Electronic Health Records: Number and Characteristics of Providers Awarded Medicare Incentive Payments for 2011-2012, GAO-14-21R (Washington, D.C.: Oct. 24, 2013); and Electronic Health Record Programs: Participation Has Increased, but Action Needed to Achieve Goals, Including Improved Quality of Care, GAO-14-207 (Washington, D.C.: Mar. 6, 2014).

[10] In this report the term stakeholders generally refers to officials we spoke with from professional associations, such as the American Medical Association, or officials from regional extension centers (REC), HIE organizations, or state public health departments.

RECs are organizations funded by the Office of the National Coordinator for Health Information Technology (ONC) to assist providers in the adoption, implementation, and meaningful use of EHRs. HITECH established the REC program, which awarded approximately $721 million in grants to create these centers. Similarly, ONC has awarded $564 million through its State Health Information Exchange Cooperative Agreement Program to states and territories to develop and advance resources to facilitate the exchange of health information among health care providers.

[11] We selected Georgia as a pilot state to test our provider interview protocol. Because the interviews in Georgia did not result in significant changes to our interview protocol, we used the results from our Georgia interviews in addition to the results from the three states we subsequently selected.

[12] The Pioneer ACO program model is an effort by the Centers for Medicare & Medicaid Services (CMS) designed to support organizations that have experience operating as ACOs in which coordinated care is delivered to beneficiaries at a lower cost to Medicare.

The Beacon Community Program consists of 17 communities throughout the country that have received funding from ONC in an effort to demonstrate how HIT investments and meaningful use of EHRs can advance the vision of patient-centered care.

[13] A health system is an organization of people, institutions, and resources that delivers health care services.

[14] 78 Fed. Reg. 14793 (March 7, 2013). CMS and ONC—both within HHS—released an RFI to seek input on a series of potential policy and programmatic changes to accelerate electronic health information exchange across providers, as well as new ideas that would be both effective and feasible to implement.

Interoperability is the ability of two or more systems or components to exchange information and to use the information that has been exchanged.

[15] GAO, Combating Terrorism: Evaluation of Selected Characteristics in National Strategies Related to Terrorism, GAO-04-408T (Washington, D.C.: Feb. 3, 2004).

[16] Pub. L. No. 103-62, 107 Stat. 285 (1993).

[17] Pub. L. No. 111-352, 124 Stat. 3866 (2011).

[18] J. Adler-Milstein and A. Jha, "Sharing Clinical Data Electronically: A Critical Challenge for Fixing the Health Care System," Journal of the American Medical Association, vol. 307, no. 16 (2012).

[19] See Pub. L. No. 111-5, § 4101(a)-(b), 123 Stat. 467-473. In 2015 the Medicare EHR program is to begin applying a payment adjustment, referred to in this report as a penalty, for hospitals and professionals that do not meet the Medicare EHR program requirements. The Medicaid EHR program does not impose penalties on Medicaid providers that do not meet the Medicaid EHR program's requirements by a specific date; however, if Medicaid providers also treat Medicare patients, they are required to meet the Medicare EHR program's requirements from 2015 onward to avoid penalties from the Medicare EHR program.

[20] See Medicare and Medicaid Programs: Electronic Health Record Incentive Program, 75 Fed. Reg. 44314 (July 28, 2010), codified at 42 C.F.R. pts. 412, 413, 422 and 495; Health Information Technology: Initial Set of Standards, Implementation Specifications, and Certification Criteria for Electronic Health Records Technology, 75 Fed. Reg. 44590 (July 28, 2010), codified at 45 C.F.R. pt. 170; Medicare and Medicaid Programs; Electronic Health Record Incentive Program—Stage 2, 77 Fed. Reg. 53968 (Sept. 4, 2012), codified at 42 C.F.R. pts. 412, 413 and 495; and Health Information Technology: Standards, Implementation Specifications, and Certification Criteria for Electronic Health Records Technology, 2014 Edition, 77 Fed. Reg. 54163 (Sept. 4, 2012), codified at 45 C.F.R. pt. 170.

[21] CMS provides states with 100 percent of the cost of incentive payments made to Medicaid providers and 90 percent of the costs related to reasonable administrative expenses and planning activities related to the Medicaid EHR program. 42 U.S.C. § 1396b(a)(3)(F)(i) and (ii).

[22] Providers can receive incentive payments from the Medicaid EHR program in their first year of participation by reporting that they adopted, implemented, or upgraded to certified EHR technology rather than demonstrating meaningful use. In subsequent years, though, they must demonstrate meaningful use to receive incentive payments.

[23] References in this report to a year in the EHR programs conform to the concept of program year, which for hospitals is based on the fiscal year and for professionals is based on the calendar year. For example, for hospitals, the 2011 program year was from October 1, 2010,

to September 30, 2011, whereas for professionals, the 2011 program year was from January 1, 2011, to December 31, 2011.

[24] Professionals do not have to satisfy this requirement if they make fewer than 100 patient transfers to another setting of care or referrals to another provider during the reporting period for the EHR programs.

[25] In general, EHR technology is not required to be certified by ONC. However, to receive EHR program incentive payments, providers must use certified EHR technology.
Health data standards are used to facilitate health information exchange and interoperability. Such standards consist of languages and technical specifications that, when adopted by multiple entities, facilitate the exchange of health information. Health data standards include, for example, standardized language for prescriptions and for laboratory testing.

[26] F. R. Goss et al., "Evaluating Standard Terminologies for Encoding Allergy Information," Journal of the American Medical Informatics Association, no. 20 (2013): 969-979. The article noted that while gaps still exist across standards related to allergies, some existing standards cover most allergy-related information.

[27] Providers who participated in the EHR programs from fiscal year 2011 through fiscal year 2013 could use certified EHR technology that conformed to the 2011 edition of the standards and certification criteria. All providers that participate in the EHR Programs in fiscal year 2014 must conform to the 2014 edition of the standards and certification criteria. ONC is expected to develop another set of standards and certification criteria that certified EHR technology would be required to conform to beginning in 2016.

[28] The CCD was created to foster interoperability of clinical data by allowing physicians to send electronic medical information to other providers. CCDs provide information such as pertinent clinical, demographic, and administrative data for a specific patient. In Stage 2, CCDs are created using consolidated clinical document architecture, which is a base standard that provides a common architecture, coding, semantic framework, and markup language for the creation of electronic clinical documents that facilitates the exchange of health information.

[29] The Direct Protocol is part of ONC's Direct Project and serves as a standard format to transmit and share clinical information necessary to satisfy some Stage 1 and Stage 2 meaningful use requirements. For example, a primary care physician who refers a patient to a specialist can use the Direct Protocol to provide a clinical summary of that patient to the specialist and receive, in return, a summary of the consultation.

[30] CMS and ONC announced in December 2013 that the agencies plan to propose a 2015 edition of the standards and certification criteria that would be voluntary for providers participating in the EHR programs. According to the agencies, this edition would respond to stakeholder feedback on the 2014 edition, and it would continue to advance health information exchange.

[31] Patient encounters are commonly recorded in free-form text narratives, or as unstructured clinical data. While free-form patient narratives give the provider flexibility to note observations that are not supported by structured data, they are not easily searchable and aggregated and can be more difficult to analyze.

[32] RxNorm, developed by HHS's National Library of Medicine, provides normalized names for clinical drugs and links its names to many of the drug vocabularies commonly used in pharmacy management and drug interaction software. SNOMED CT is a set of clinical terminology owned and maintained by the International Health Terminology Standards Development Organisation. RxNorm and SNOMED CT are examples of standards that are required by the 2014 edition of the standards and certification criteria.

[33] HHS officials stated that the Direct Protocol could be used to enable more sophisticated means of exchange, such as alerts to providers when patients are admitted to a hospital. However, the availability of these features varies by EHR vendor and geographic location.

[34] HIPAA's Administrative Simplification Provisions required the establishment of, among other things, national privacy standards. Pub. L. No. 104-191, Title II, Subtitle F, 110 Stat. 1936, 2021 (codified at 42 U.S.C. §§ 1320d–1320d-8). These provisions also expressly provided that such national standards would not preempt state laws that impose requirements, standards, or implementation specifications that are more stringent than those imposed under federal regulation. Pub. L. No. 104-191, Title II, Subtitle F, 110 Stat. 1936, 2021, see 42 U.S.C. §§ 1320d–2 notes. HIPAA regulates covered entities' (including most health care providers') use and disclosure of personal health information. The Privacy Rule generally permits the use or disclosure of an individual's protected health information without the individual's written authorization for purposes of treatment, payment and health care operations. Under the Privacy Rule, more stringent state laws that are not preempted by federal law include those that prohibit or restrict a use or disclosure in circumstances under which such use or disclosure would be permitted under HIPAA. See 45 C.F.R. 160.202.

[35] Data segmentation is a process that enables the sharing of some but not all health information. According to researchers, data segmentation could enable patient control over the sharing or withholding of health information.

[36] Audacious Inquiry, LLC, Patient Identification and Matching Final Report, a report prepared at the request of the Department of Health and Human Services, Office of the National Coordinator for Health Information Technology, Feb. 7, 2014.

[37] U.S. Department of Health and Human Services, Health IT Policy Committee letter to the National Coordinator for Health Information Technology, February 8, 2011, accessed September 10, 2013, http://healthit.hhs.gov/portal/server.pt/community/ healthit_hhs_gov__policy_recommendati ons/1815. U.S. Department of Health and Human Services, Health IT Standards Committee letter to the National Coordinator for Health Information Technology, August 17, 2011, accessed December 31, 2013, http://www.healthit.gov/policy-researchers-implementers/health-it-standards-committee-recommendations-national-coordinator-h.

[38] HHS has stated that it is prohibited from implementing a national patient identifier and referred to the Omnibus Consolidated and Emergency Supplemental Appropriations Act of 1999. The act prohibits HHS from using any funds to promulgate or adopt any final standard providing for, or providing for the assignment of, a unique health identifier for an individual until legislation is enacted specifically approving the standard. See Pub. L. No. 105-277, § 516, 112 Stat. 2681, 2681-386 (1998).

[39] ONC's State Health Information Exchange Cooperative Agreement Program has provided funding for 56 states, eligible territories, and qualified State Designated Entities since March 2010.

ONC officials also stated that the Direct Protocol is a low-cost option for exchanging health information, and therefore may help providers reduce the cost of exchanging health information.

[40] Two states, Florida and Ohio, requested to end their funding support from ONC's State Health Information Exchange Cooperative Agreement Program in fall 2013, according to ONC officials.

[41] J. Adler-Milstein, D. W. Bates, and A. K. Jha, "Operational Health Information Exchanges Show Substantial Growth, but Long-Term Funding Remains a Concern," Health Affairs, vol. 32, no. 8 (2013).

[42] The requirement to provide a summary of care document for each transition of care or referral in Stage 2 also requires eligible professionals and hospitals to provide summary of care documents for more than 10 percent of transitions of care and referrals either (1) electronically transmitted using certified EHR technology or (2) through an exchange with an organization that is a Nationwide Health Information Network Exchange participant or in a way that is consistent with the Nationwide Health Information Network. The Nationwide Health Information Network was a program funded by ONC that transitioned to the eHealth Exchange, a group of federal agencies and nonfederal organizations whose mission, among other things, is to improve public health reporting through secure, trusted, and interoperable health information exchange.

CMS and ONC have identified a minimum set of technical capabilities that are required for an EHR to be considered a test EHR. Eligible professionals and hospitals that select to attest to this requirement will be randomly matched with a designated test EHR that is designed by an EHR developer other than the sender's.

[43]For more information, see the Department of Health and Human Services, the Office of the National Coordinator for Health Information Technology, and the Centers for Medicare & Medicaid Services, Principles and Strategy for Accelerating Health Information Exchange (HIE), (Aug. 7, 2013).

[44] GAO-04-408T.

See Pub L. No. 103-62, 107 Stat. 285 (1993) (GPRA), as amended by Pub. L. No. 111- 352, 124 Stat. 3866 (2011) (GPRAMA). GPRA requires, among other things, that federal agencies develop strategic plans that include agencywide goals and strategies for achieving those goals. We have reported that these requirements also can serve as leading practices for planning at lower levels within federal agencies, such as individual programs or initiatives.

[45] GAO, Agency Performance Plans: Examples of Practices That Can Improve Usefulness to Decisionmakers, GAO/GGD/AIMD-99-69 (Washington, D.C.: Feb. 26, 1999), and GAO, Executive Guide: Effectively Implementing the Government Performance and Results Act, GAO/GGD-96-118 (Washington, D.C.: June 1996).

End Notes for Appendix I

[1] The Continuity of Care Document (CCD) was created to foster interoperability of clinical data by allowing physicians to send electronic medical information to other providers. The purpose of the CCD is to allow the transmission of information without loss of clinical meaning. CCDs provide information such as pertinent clinical, demographic, and administrative data for a specific patient.

[2] The Direct Protocol is part of the Office of the National Coordinator for Health Information Technology's (ONC) Direct Project and serves as a standard format to transmit and share clinical information necessary to satisfy some Stage 1 and Stage 2 meaningful use requirements for the EHR programs. For example, a primary care physician who refers a patient to a specialist can use the Direct Protocol to provide a clinical summary of that patient to the specialist and receive, in return, a summary of the consultation.

[3] Interoperability is the ability of two or more systems or components to exchange information and use the information that has been exchanged.

[4] See 2012 Mass. Acts. ch. 224 (August 6, 2012).

End Note for Appendix III

[1] For more information, see Office of the National Coordinator for Health Information Technology and the Centers for Medicare & Medicaid Services, Principles and Strategy for Accelerating Health Information Exchange (HIE). August 7, 2013.

INDEX

A

abstraction, 15, 16, 31, 67
access, 4, 9, 11, 14, 25, 26, 27, 45, 46, 49, 53, 56, 60, 64, 69, 70, 78, 97, 98, 101, 104, 105
accountability, 14, 16, 28, 78, 88, 90
adjustment, 4, 35, 107
advancement, 73
adverse event, 71
age, 44, 47, 48, 63
agencies, 8, 16, 24, 25, 28, 30, 31, 32, 33, 34, 35, 36, 37, 48, 50, 53, 56, 71, 77, 86, 90, 91, 92, 101, 103, 108, 110
allergic reaction, 84, 86
allergy, 26, 27, 43, 44, 45, 52, 84, 94, 108
American Recovery and Reinvestment Act, 4, 63, 76, 79
American Recovery and Reinvestment Act of 2009, 4, 63, 76, 79
Appropriations Act, 109
Appropriations Committee, 71, 73
assessment, 87
assets, 9
audit(s), 8, 72, 81

B

barriers, 9, 35
base, 108
beneficiaries, 63, 67, 71, 106
benefits, 62, 71, 89, 94, 96, 97
blood, 27, 44
blood pressure, 27, 44
bonuses, 64

C

cancer, 49, 50, 64, 70, 102
certification, 5, 12, 28, 29, 30, 37, 66, 70, 83, 84, 85, 88, 92, 93, 108
challenges, viii, 2, 5, 9, 25, 28, 36, 76, 77, 79, 80, 84, 87, 88, 90, 91, 92, 103
children, 44, 64
clarity, 86
coding, 108
communication, 79
communities, 63, 107
community, 59, 96, 109
compliance, 45
computation, 70
Congress, 4
Congressional Budget Office, 4, 38, 64, 106
consent, 86, 87, 105
constituents, 104
consumers, 104
coordination, 5, 67, 78, 79, 83, 88, 92, 104
cost, 9, 64, 88, 89, 106, 107, 109
covering, 77, 86, 88
CT, 76, 86, 108

D

data analysis, 8
data collection, 15, 24, 67
deficiencies, 12, 46
demographic data, 88
Department of Health and Human Services, 2, 3, 5, 58, 71, 73, 75, 77, 79, 104, 109, 110
diabetes, 34, 70
directives, 48, 53, 56
discharges, 9
disclosure, 109
diseases, 70, 94
District of Columbia, 39, 64, 65, 68
doctors, 10, 19, 21, 50, 64, 72
draft, 37, 76, 93
drug interaction, vii, 1, 108
drugs, vii, 1, 108

E

early warning, 16
education, 47, 53, 55, 64
educational materials, 22
EHR data, vii, 1, 6, 7
EHR technology, vii, viii, 1, 4, 5, 9, 11, 12, 30, 36, 37, 42, 46, 47, 48, 49, 50, 58, 59, 64, 66, 76, 77, 79, 81, 83, 84, 85, 96, 106, 107, 108, 110
emergency, 69, 97
employment, 17
encoding, 84
encryption, 46
end-stage renal disease, 63
ethnicity, 27, 44
evidence, 8, 23, 25, 38, 69, 81
exclusion, 65
expenditures, 4, 5, 83

F

facilitators, 81
federal advisory, 87
federal government, 5, 104
federal law, 109
financial, 15, 71
financial incentives, 15
flexibility, 50, 53, 56, 108
food, 73
funding, 4, 5, 69, 79, 82, 83, 89, 93, 107, 109
funds, 63, 109

G

GAO, vii, viii, 1, 2, 3, 17, 18, 19, 20, 27, 50, 53, 56, 60, 61, 62, 64, 65, 66, 67, 69, 70, 71, 75, 76, 77, 82, 103, 105, 106, 107, 110
Georgia, 80, 94, 95, 96, 106
GPRA, 75, 81, 110
grants, 64, 69, 106
growth, 15, 44, 61, 79, 81
guidance, vii, 2, 3, 8, 16, 22, 27, 32, 34, 36, 50, 53, 56, 86, 88, 93, 103, 104

H

hazards, 71
Health and Human Services, 36, 92, 106, 109
health care, 3, 4, 5, 6, 12, 15, 16, 32, 33, 34, 35, 36, 37, 38, 61, 63, 73, 78, 79, 83, 89, 92, 93, 96, 106, 107, 109
health care costs, 4, 15, 38, 61
health care professionals, 83
health care system, 63, 73, 78, 92
health condition, 45, 105
Health Information Technology for Economic and Clinical Health Act, vii, 10, 64, 76, 79, 106
health insurance, 6, 38, 63, 71
height, 27, 44
HHS, v, vii, viii, 1, 2, 3, 5, 7, 8, 12, 15, 16, 28, 31, 32, 33, 35, 37, 58, 60, 61, 66, 67, 70, 73, 75, 76, 77, 79, 80, 83, 84, 85, 87,

88, 89, 90, 91, 92, 93, 94, 104, 105, 106, 107, 108, 109
higher education, 64
history, 49, 97
HITECH, vii, 1, 4, 5, 11, 12, 37, 38, 63, 76, 79, 82, 88, 105, 106
HIV, 105
homes, 34
human, 87
human immunodeficiency virus, 87

I

identification, 24
images, 49, 102
immunization, 25, 48, 56, 70, 94, 100
improvements, 16, 34, 36, 37, 63, 77, 78, 85, 91
incentive payments, vii, viii, 1, 2, 4, 5, 6, 9, 10, 11, 13, 18, 19, 20, 21, 23, 28, 39, 40, 42, 51, 59, 60, 63, 64, 65, 66, 67, 68, 69, 70, 72, 76, 83, 107, 108
income, 63
individuals, 6, 16, 28, 63, 73
industry, 38
information exchange, viii, 14, 28, 59, 76, 77, 78, 79, 80, 81, 84, 88, 90, 93, 94, 97, 103, 104, 105
information sharing, 63
information technology, 61, 63, 104
infrastructure, 11, 12, 61, 63
institutions, 64, 107
integration, 105
integrity, 90, 104
interoperability, 28, 66, 80, 84, 90, 95, 103, 104, 108, 110
investment(s), 5, 34, 63, 107
issues, 3, 30, 35, 36, 37, 66, 70, 77, 84, 86, 87

J

job training, 17
jurisdiction, 79

L

languages, 108
laws, 86, 87, 109
lead, 14, 30, 67, 77, 78, 85, 89, 90, 91, 92, 103
learning, 73
legend, 18
legislation, 38, 109

M

magnitude, 5
majority, 33
management, 14, 16, 86, 91, 105, 108
market share, 71
mass, 27, 44
materials, 7, 22, 28
measurement, 3, 7, 28, 30, 31, 35, 66, 105
median, 66
medical, 5, 15, 31, 32, 34, 38, 42, 64, 66, 71, 73, 97, 108, 110
medical care, 66, 97
medication, 23, 24, 26, 27, 43, 44, 45, 47, 49, 52, 53, 54, 55, 57, 66, 81, 94, 95, 97, 98, 99, 102
medicine, 10, 11, 19, 21, 50, 64, 72
mental health, 87
messages, 85
mission(s), 16, 28, 35, 110
models, 79
modifications, 31
mortality, 44

N

narratives, 85, 108
natural disaster, 11

O

obstacles, 28, 30

officials, vii, viii, 2, 6, 7, 8, 16, 21, 22, 30, 31, 34, 39, 50, 51, 53, 54, 56, 57, 61, 69, 70, 76, 80, 81, 84, 85, 86, 87, 89, 90, 91, 92, 94, 95, 97, 103, 106, 109
operations, 17, 109
opportunities, 35, 77, 89
osteopathy, 64
outpatient, 71
outreach, 22, 46
oversight, 78, 90

P

participants, 17, 62
patient care, 42, 62, 85, 96
peer review, 61, 62
penalties, vii, 1, 2, 9, 10, 11, 15, 17, 21, 64, 66, 68, 69, 83, 107
performance measurement, 63
performance rate, 31
permit, 56
physicians, viii, 2, 4, 7, 25, 41, 58, 59, 62, 64, 76, 80, 81, 83, 105, 108, 110
policy, 37, 66, 93, 107, 109
population, 16, 42, 61, 62, 67
principles, 76, 77, 90, 91, 93, 103
private sector, 38, 71, 93
program outcomes, 3, 33, 58, 60
project, 87
public health, 24, 25, 48, 49, 56, 67, 70, 71, 81, 94, 97, 101, 102, 105, 106, 110

Q

quality improvement, 14, 28, 31, 46
query, 86

R

race, 27, 44
recommendations, 2, 5, 37, 66, 76, 88, 93, 109
reconciliation, 24, 47, 53, 55, 99
reform(s), 34, 36, 38, 93, 104
registries, 25, 48, 56, 67, 100
regulations, vii, 2, 6, 7, 27, 66, 104
relatives, 49
reliability, 2, 3, 8, 28, 30, 31, 35, 36, 37, 39, 41, 71
requirements, vii, 1, 2, 3, 4, 5, 7, 8, 9, 10, 11, 12, 14, 16, 17, 22, 23, 26, 27, 30, 33, 34, 35, 36, 38, 39, 51, 63, 65, 66, 67, 68, 70, 71, 72, 73, 81, 83, 86, 87, 89, 92, 97, 103, 104, 107, 108, 109, 110
researchers, 109
resources, 47, 53, 55, 67, 87, 88, 106, 107
response, 66, 85
revenue, 42
rewards, 15
risk(s), 14, 28, 34, 35, 46, 66, 88, 92
rules, 73, 77, 84, 86
rural areas, 22, 63

S

safety, 3, 5, 6, 32, 33, 34, 35, 36, 37, 58, 60, 61, 67, 71, 73, 78, 87, 91, 92
savings, 38
scientific knowledge, 73
scope, 69
security, 46, 86, 90, 104, 106
services, 11, 17, 63, 64, 66, 69, 78, 79, 103, 105, 107
sex, 27, 44
sexually transmitted infections, 87
shortage, 66
signs, 24, 27, 44, 52, 54
smoking, 24, 27, 44, 52, 54
Social Security, 64
socioeconomic background, 104
software, 9, 108
specifications, 28, 29, 30, 35, 36, 70, 83, 106, 108, 109
speculation, 38
spending, 4, 38, 64, 78, 79
stakeholder groups, vii, 2
stakeholders, viii, 6, 28, 76, 77, 79, 80, 81, 82, 84, 86, 87, 88, 89, 90, 91, 94, 95, 103, 106

state borders, 86
state laws, 86, 109
statutes, vii, 2
structure, 105
suppliers, 105
surveillance, 24, 25, 29, 48, 56, 101

T

target, 33
technical comments, 93
techniques, 67
technologies, 49
technology, vii, viii, 1, 4, 5, 9, 11, 12, 29, 30, 36, 37, 38, 42, 46, 47, 48, 49, 50, 58, 59, 61, 63, 64, 66, 73, 76, 77, 78, 79, 81, 83, 84, 85, 89, 96, 99, 100, 101, 102, 106, 107, 108, 110
testing, 8, 12, 29, 30, 36, 37, 39, 70, 86, 97, 108
time frame, 76, 78, 90, 91, 92, 93
Title I, 109
Title II, 109
training, 28, 63, 87
transmission, 81, 85, 110
treatment, 28, 78, 109

U

unforeseen circumstances, 11
United States, v, 1, 63, 67, 75
urban, 69
urban areas, 69

V

validation, 32
variations, 86
vision, 107

W

Washington, 64, 65, 67, 71, 72, 73, 106, 107, 110
web, 15, 96
workflow, 30
workforce, 63